MICHIGAN STATE UNIVI
LIBRARY
WITHDRAWN

D0275963

**V** VETERINARY

**M** MEDICAL

**S** SCHOOL

**A** ADMISSION

**R** REQUIREMENTS

*in the*

*United States*

*and Canada*

MICHIGAN STATE UNIVERSITY
LIBRARY
WITHDRAWN

# VETERINARY MEDICAL SCHOOL ADMISSION REQUIREMENTS

## in the
## United States and Canada

*2001 Edition for 2002 Matriculation*

Association of American
Veterinary Medical Colleges

PURDUE UNIVERSITY PRESS          WEST LAFAYETTE, INDIANA

VET MED CTR
LIB

SF
776
.N7
V47
2001

Copyright ©2001 by the Association of American Veterinary
Medical Colleges. All rights reserved.

∞™ The paper used in this book meets the minimum requirements
of American National Standard for Information Sciences—
Permanence of Paper for Printed Library Materials, ANSI Z39.48-1992.

Cover photo: *Continuum,* an original bronze sculpture by artist Larry Anderson, of Boney Lake,
Washington, was dedicated at the Purdue University School of Veterinary Medicine on September 23,
2000. Photograph by Dr. Dennis DeNicola, professor of veterinary pathobiology, Purdue University.

Printed in the United States of America

ISBN 1-55753-229-X
ISSN 1089-6465

# CONTENTS

# Foreword

The opportunities and options for veterinarians are more varied than ever. Today's veterinary student can choose to train for a career in environmental problem-solving, local community health, food resource management, zoo animal care, space and marine biology, or wildlife preservation in addition to the more traditional small- or large-animal practice.

The choices begin with selecting and applying to the right veterinary medical schools. An uninformed decision could lead to costly mistakes, or even academic failure. Students, parents, mentors, and counselors need help to make sure that such important decisions are based on sound knowledge, and *Veterinary Medical School Admission Requirements (VMSAR)* is an invaluable source for this essential information.

This 17th edition provides current information for all thirty-one veterinary medical schools in the United States and Canada. The entry for each school includes information on the admissions office contact, prerequisite courses, application deadlines, standardized test requirements, residency implications, timetables, cost of education, and other admission policies and procedures. This book also includes information on special programs, statistical data on the national applicant pool, and minority student opportunities. A valuable new feature, "Financing Your Veterinary Medical Education," was provided by Deb Burdick, assistant director at Iowa State University's Office of Student Financial Aid.

VMSAR is compiled annually under the auspices of the Association of American Veterinary Medical Colleges (AAVMC). The AAVMC welcomes suggestions for future editions; they may be directed to Denise A. Ottinger, Director of Student Services, 1240 Lynn Hall, School of Veterinary Medicine, Purdue University, West Lafayette, Indiana 47907-1240.

My thanks to each of the veterinary medical schools for their assistance in making this book possible each year.

Denise A. Ottinger, Editor
*School of Veterinary Medicine at Purdue University*

# ABBREVIATIONS

| | |
|---|---|
| AAVMC | Association of American Veterinary Medical Colleges |
| AVMA | American Veterinary Medical Association |
| BA/BS | Bachelor of Arts or Bachelor of Science degrees |
| CVMA | Canadian Veterinary Medical Association |
| DVM/VMD | Doctor of Veterinary Medicine degree |
| GRE | Graduate Record Examination |
| MCAT | Medical College Admission Test |
| MS | Master of Science degree |
| PhD | Doctor of Philosophy degree |
| SREB | Southern Regional Education Board |
| TOEFL | Test of English as a Foreign Language |
| VCAT | Veterinary College Admission Test |
| VMCAS | Veterinary Medical College Application Service |
| VMD/DVM | Veterinary Medical Doctor degree |
| VMSAR | Veterinary Medical School Admission Requirements |
| WICHE | Western Interstate Commission for Higher Education |

# Veterinary Medicine: Choices and Challenges

Considered from the perspective of comparative medicine, veterinarians help animals and people live longer, healthier lives. They serve society by preventing and treating animal disease, improving the quality of the environment, ensuring the safety of food, controlling diseases transmitted from animals, and advancing medical knowledge. The Doctor of Veterinary Medicine degree can lead to diverse career opportunities and different lifestyles from a solo mixed-animal practice in a rural area to a teaching or research position at an urban university, medical center, or industrial laboratory. The majority of veterinarians in the United States are in private practice, although significant numbers are involved in preventive medicine, regulatory veterinary medicine, military veterinary medicine, laboratory animal medicine, research and development in industry, and teaching and research in a variety of basic science and clinical disciplines.

## License to Practice

The DVM (or VMD) degree is awarded after 4 years of successful study at an accredited college of veterinary medicine. Graduate veterinarians are eligible to apply for a license to practice. Licensing is controlled by states and provinces, each of which has rules and procedures for legal practice within its own jurisdiction. All require satisfactory completion of the national board examination, and most have other requirements, including additional tests and interviews.

## Specialization

Graduate veterinarians may choose to become specialists in a clinical area or to work with particular species. The first step on the path toward specialization is usually an internship.

## Internship

Internships are 1-year programs in either small- or large-animal medicine and surgery. The most prestigious internship programs are at veterinary medical colleges or at very large private veterinary hospitals with board-certified veterinarians on staff. Since internships are usually at large referral centers, interns are exposed to a larger number of challenging cases than they would be likely to see in a smaller private practice.

Veterinary students in their senior year and veterinary graduates apply for

1

internships through a matching program. Internship applicants and training hospitals rank each other in order of preference, and a computerized system matches each applicant with the highest-ranking teaching hospital that ranked the applicant. Academic performance in the veterinary professional curriculum, as well as recommendations from veterinary school faculty, is considered in the ranking of internship applicants.

Most veterinary interns in the United States receive a nominal salary, and their educational debts, if any, may be postponed in some governmentally subsidized loan programs. Veterinarians can often command a higher starting salary in private practice after completion of an internship. Also, an internship is the next step, after receiving the DVM degree, toward residency and board certification.

## Residency Training

Veterinarians who complete internships or who have 2 years of private-practice experience are eligible to apply for residency programs. Residency training is more specialized than an internship. Currently, residency training is available in internal medicine, surgery, cardiology, dermatology, ophthalmology, exotic small animal medicine, pathology, neurology, radiology, anesthesiology, and oncology. The programs take 2 to 3 years to complete, depending on the nature of the specialty. Successful completion of a residency is required for certification by any of the veterinary medical specialty boards. Some residencies combine research and graduate study to lead to a master's degree.

## Board Certification

Veterinary board certification and diplomate status are available for 20 specialties: anesthesiology, animal behavior, clinical pharmacology, dentistry, dermatology, emergency and critical care, internal medicine, laboratory animal medicine, microbiology, nutrition, ophthalmology, pathology, poultry medicine, private practice, preventive medicine, radiology, surgery, theriogenology (reproduction), toxicology, and zoological medicine.

## Private and Public Practice

A significant percentage of veterinary graduates are engaged in private practice, either as an owner of a solo practice or, more likely, as a partner or associate in a group practice. Increasingly, veterinarians work together as a team, which allows a wider range of services to be provided.

Small-animal veterinarians focus their efforts primarily on dogs and cats but are seeing a growing number of pet birds and exotic animals such as reptiles.

Veterinarians specializing in large animals often place their emphasis on horses, cattle, or pigs, and work both on a farm-call and an in-clinic basis. A mixed-animal veterinarian works with all types of animals.

Some veterinarians obtain further specialization in such areas as diseases or disorders of the eyes of cats or reproduction difficulties in cattle.

Public practice provides a variety of opportunities at the national, state, county, or city levels. Opportunities in food safety, public health, the military, animal disease control, research, and the care and maintenance of wildlife abound.

## Industry

Veterinarians have many opportunities available to them in private industry, particularly in the fields of nutrition and pharmaceuticals. Assisting in the development of new products in the animal industry, conducting research for pharmaceutical companies, diagnosing disease and drug effects as pathologists, or safeguarding the health of laboratory animal colonies are all interesting career possibilities. Some veterinarians may be employed by zoos and aquariums and may act as consultants to wildlife preservation groups, game farms, or fisheries.

## New or Unusual Career Opportunities

By the very nature of the many species of animals involved and the wide variety of clientele served, the opportunities available to today's veterinarian are abundant. The role of the veterinarian in society has changed and evolved over time, so that they are now specially qualified to take part in many problems related to the environment, local community health, food resource management, zoo animal care, space and marine biology, and wildlife preservation.

Residents of the Exotic Feline Rescue Center in Center Point, Indiana, are frequent patients at the University of Illinois College of Veterinary Medicine. Photo by Lil Morales, courtesy of the University of Illinois College of Veterinary Medicine.

# Alphabetical Listing of Veterinary Schools

**United States**

| | |
|---|---|
| Auburn University | Auburn University, Alabama |
| California, University of | Davis, California |
| Colorado State University | Fort Collins, Colorado |
| Cornell University | Ithaca, New York |
| Florida, University of | Gainesville, Florida |
| Georgia, University of | Athens, Georgia |
| Illinois, University of | Urbana, Illinois |
| Iowa State University | Ames, Iowa |
| Kansas State University | Manhattan, Kansas |
| Louisiana State University | Baton Rouge, Louisiana |
| Michigan State University | East Lansing, Michigan |
| Minnesota, University of | St. Paul, Minnesota |
| Mississippi State University | Mississippi State, Mississippi |
| Missouri, University of | Columbia, Missouri |
| North Carolina State University | Raleigh, North Carolina |
| Ohio State University | Columbus, Ohio |
| Oklahoma State University | Stillwater, Oklahoma |
| Oregon State University | Corvallis, Oregon |
| Pennsylvania, University of | Philadelphia, Pennsylvania |
| Purdue University | West Lafayette, Indiana |
| Tennessee, University of | Knoxville, Tennessee |
| Texas A & M University | College Station, Texas |
| Tufts University | North Grafton, Massachusetts |
| Tuskegee University | Tuskegee, Alabama |
| Virginia Polytechnic Institute and State University (Virginia-Maryland Regional) | Blacksburg, Virginia |
| Washington State University | Pullman, Washington |
| Wisconsin, University of | Madison, Wisconsin |

**Canada**

| | |
|---|---|
| Guelph, University of | Guelph, Ontario |
| Montréal, Université de | Montréal, Québec |
| Prince Edward Island, University of | Charlottetown, Prince Edward Island |
| Saskatchewan, University of | Saskatoon, Saskatchewan |

# GEOGRAPHICAL LISTING OF VETERINARY SCHOOLS AND DIRECTORY OF ADMISSIONS OFFICES

## United States

### Alabama

Office for Academic Affairs
College of Veterinary Medicine
217 Goodwin Student Center
Auburn University
Auburn University AL 36849-5536

College of Veterinary Medicine,
    Nursing, and Allied Health
Tuskegee University
Tuskegee AL 36088

### California

Office of the Dean-Student Programs
School of Veterinary Medicine
One Shields Avenue
University of California
Davis CA 95616

### Colorado

Office of the Dean
College of Veterinary Medicine and
    Biomedical Sciences
Colorado State University
Fort Collins CO 80523-1601

### Florida

Admissions Office
College of Veterinary Medicine
P.O. Box 100125
University of Florida
Gainesville FL 32610-0125

### Georgia

Office for Academic Affairs
College of Veterinary Medicine
The University of Georgia
Athens GA 30602-7372

### Illinois

Office of Academic and Student
    Affairs
College of Veterinary Medicine
University of Illinois at Urbana-
    Champaign
2271G Veterinary Medicine Basic
    Sciences Bldg.
2001 South Lincoln Avenue
Urbana IL 61802

### Indiana

Student Services Office
School of Veterinary Medicine
1240 Lynn Hall
Purdue University
West Lafayette IN 47907-1240

### Iowa

Office of Admissions
College of Veterinary Medicine
2524 Veterinary Medicince
Iowa State University
Ames IA 50011-1250

**Kansas**
Office of Admissions
College of Veterinary Medicine
101 Trotter Hall
1700 Denison Avenue
Kansas State University
Manhattan KS 66506-5601

**Louisiana**
Office of Veterinary Student and
    Academic Affairs
School of Veterinary Medicine
Louisiana State University
Baton Rouge LA 70803

**Massachusetts**
Office of Admissions
School of Veterinary Medicine
200 Westboro Road
Tufts University
North Grafton MA 01536

**Michigan**
Office of Admissions
College of Veterinary Medicine
A-126 East Fee Hall
Michigan State University
East Lansing MI 48824-1316

**Minnesota**
Office of Student Affairs and
    Admissions
College of Veterinary Medicine
460 Veterinary Teaching Hospital
1365 Gortner Avenue
University of Minnesota
St. Paul MN 55108

**Mississippi**
Office of Student Affairs
College of Veterinary Medicine
P.O. Box 9825
Mississippi State University
Mississippi State MS 39762

**Missouri**
Office of Academic Affairs
College of Veterinary Medicine
W203 Veterinary Medicine Building
University of Missouri-Columbia
Columbia MO 65211

**New York**
Office of DVM Admissions
College of Veterinary Medicine
S2-009 Schurman Hall
Cornell University
Ithaca NY 14853-6401

**North Carolina**
Student Services Office
College of Veterinary Medicine
4700 Hillsborough Street
North Carolina State University
Raleigh NC 27606

**Ohio**
Chairperson, Admissions Committee
College of Veterinary Medicine
0004 Veterinary Hospital
601 Tharp Street
The Ohio State University
Columbus OH 43210-1089

**Oklahoma**
Admissions Office
College of Veterinary Medicine
Oklahoma State University
Stillwater OK 74078-2003

**Oregon**
Office of the Dean
College of Veterinary Medicine
Oregon State University
200 Magruder Hall
Corvallis OR 97331-4801

**Pennsylvania**
Admissions Office
School of Veterinary Medicine
3800 Spruce Street
University of Pennsylvania
Philadelphia PA 19104-6044

**Tennessee**
Office of the Associate Dean
College of Veterinary Medicine
P.O. Box 1071
University of Tennessee
Knoxville TN 37901-1071

**Texas**
Office of the Dean
College of Veterinary Medicine
Texas A & M University
College Station TX 77843-4461

**Virginia**
Admissions Coordinator
Virginia-Maryland Regional College
of Veterinary Medicine
Virginia Polytechnic Institute and
State University
Blacksburg VA 24061

**Washington**
Office of Student Services
College of Veterinary Medicine
Washington State University
Pullman WA 99164-7012

**Wisconsin**
Office of Academic Affairs
School of Veterinary Medicine
2015 Linden Drive West
University of Wisconsin-Madison
Madison WI 53706-1102

## Canada

**Montréal**
Service des Admissions
Université de Montréal
C.P. 6205
Succursale Centre-Ville
Montréal Québec H3C 3T5

**Ontario**
Admissions, Office of Registrarial
Services
University Centre, Level 3
University of Guelph
Guelph Ontario N1G 2W1

**Prince Edward Island**
Registrar's Office
Atlantic Veterinary College
University of Prince Edward Island
550 University Avenue
Charlottetown PEI C1A 4P3

**Saskatchewan**
Admissions Office
Western College of Veterinary
    Medicine
University of Saskatchewan
52 Campus Drive
Saskatoon Saskatchewan S7N 5B4

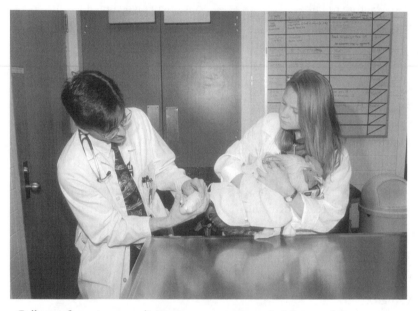

Colleges of veterinary medicine encourage teamwork. Here, students prepare to examine a chicken's injured foot. Photo by Phil Snow, courtesy of the University of Tennessee College of Veterinary Medicine.

# Listing of Schools Accepting Nonresident/Noncontract Applications

| United States | Number of Positions Available |
|---|---|
| Auburn University | 10 positions; U.S. citizens only. |
| University of California | Limited number of positions. |
| Colorado State University | Up to 20 positions; international applicants considered. |
| Cornell University | Up to 30 positions; international applicants considered. |
| University of Florida | Not more than 15% of entering class. |
| University of Georgia | Up to 10 positions. |
| University of Illinois | 20 positions. |
| Iowa State University | Up to 25 positions, plus unfilled contract positions; international applicants considered. |
| Kansas State University | 15-20% of class, plus unfilled contract positions; international applicants considered. |
| Louisiana State University | Up to 15 positions. |
| Michigan State University | Not more than 20-25% of entering class; international applicants considered. |
| University of Minnesota | Not more than 25% of entering class. |
| Mississippi State University | Up to 19 positions. |
| University of Missouri | 10 positions. |
| North Carolina State University | 12 positions. |
| Ohio State University | Up to 35 positions. |
| Oklahoma State University | Up to 14 positions. |

| | |
|---|---|
| Oregon State University | Up to 8 positions. |
| University of Pennsylvania | 45–50 positions; international applicants considered. |
| Purdue University | 20 positions; international applicants considered. |
| University of Tennessee | Limited number of positions. |
| Texas A & M University | Up to 10 positions. |
| Tufts University | Up to 40 positions. |
| Tuskegee University | Up to 10 positions; international applicants considered. |
| Virginia-Maryland Regional College of Veterinary Medicine | Up to 10 positions. |
| Washington State University | Limited number of positions. |
| University of Wisconsin | Up to 20 positions. |

**Canada**

| | |
|---|---|
| University of Prince Edward Island | 19 positions for international applicants. |

# Listing of Contracting States and Provinces

All Canadian provinces and 20 states in the United States that do not have a veterinary school contract with one or more schools to provide access to veterinary medical education for their residents. The state or province, working through the contracting agency, usually agrees to pay a fee to help cover the cost of education for a certain number of places in each entering class. Residents from the contract states then compete with each other for those positions.

Some states contract with more than one school. For example, Arkansas contracts with 5 veterinary schools, and North Dakota has contracts with 6 schools. Connecticut, Rhode Island, Vermont, and the District of Columbia presently have no contracts, so all candidates from these places apply as nonresidents to veterinary schools of their choice.

The educational agreements between contracting agencies and veterinary schools differ. Under some contract arrangements, students pay in-state tuition; in others, they pay nonresident tuition. Some contract states require students to repay all or part of the subsidy that the state provided; others require veterinary graduates to return to practice in the state for a period of time. Applicants should be aware of their obligation to the state before agreeing to participate in a contract program.

Following is a list of states and provinces that have educational agreements with schools of veterinary medicine.

## UNITED STATES

### Alaska
Contracts through WICHE* with University of California, Colorado State University, Oregon State University, and Washington State University.

### Arizona
Contracts through WICHE* with University of California, Colorado State University, Oregon State University, and Washington State University.

### Arkansas
Contracts in past with Tuskegee University, Louisiana State University, University of Missouri, and Oklahoma State University. Contracts not all completed at time of printing; may be some changes.

### Delaware
Contracts with Virginia-Maryland Regional College.

* WICHE = Western Interstate Commission for Higher Education (offices in Boulder, Colorado)

11

### Georgia
Contracts with Tuskegee University, in addition to having a school in the state.

### Hawaii
Contracts through WICHE* with University of California, Colorado State University, Oregon State University, and Washington State University.

### Idaho
Contracts with Washington State University.

### Kentucky
Contracts with Auburn University and Tuskegee University.

### Maine
Contracts with Tufts University.

### Montana
Contracts through WICHE* with University of California, Colorado State University, Oregon State University, and Washington State University.

### Nebraska
Contracts with Kansas State University.

### Nevada
Contracts through WICHE* with University of California, Colorado State University, Oregon State University, and Washington State University.

### New Hampshire
Contracts with Cornell University and Tufts University.

### New Jersey
Contracts with Cornell University, University of Illinois, Iowa State University, University of Pennsylvania, Oklahoma State University, Tufts University, and Tuskegee University.

### New Mexico
Contracts through WICHE* with University of California, Colorado State University, Oregon State University, and Washington State University.

### North Dakota
Reciprocity with University of Minnesota. Contracts with Iowa State University. Contracts through WICHE* with University of California, Colorado State University, Oregon State University, and Washington State University.

* WICHE = Western Interstate Commission for Higher Education (offices in Boulder, Colorado)

**Puerto Rico**
Contracts with Tuskegee University. Cooperative agreement with University of Wisconsin.

**South Carolina**
Contracts with University of Georgia and Tuskegee University.

**South Dakota**
Reciprocity with University of Minnesota. Contracts with Iowa State University.

**Utah**
Contracts through WICHE* with University of California, Colorado State University, Oregon State University, and Washington State University.

**West Virginia**
Contracts with University of Georgia, Ohio State University, and Tuskegee University.

**Wyoming**
Contracts through WICHE* with the University of California, Colorado State University, Oregon State University, and Washington State University.

# CANADA

**Alberta**
Contracts with University of Saskatchewan.

**British Columbia**
Contracts with University of Saskatchewan.

**Manitoba**
Reciprocity with University of Minnesota. Contracts with University of Saskatchewan.

**New Brunswick**
Contracts with Atlantic Veterinary College at the University of Prince Edward Island and Université de Montréal.

**Newfoundland**
Contracts with Atlantic Veterinary College at the University of Prince Edward Island.

**Nova Scotia**
Contracts with Atlantic Veterinary College at the University of Prince Edward Island.

**Yukon Territory**
Contracts with University of Saskatchewan.

* WICHE = Western Interstate Commission for Higher Education (offices in Boulder, Colorado)

# Programs for Multicultural or Disadvantaged Students

The Association of American Veterinary Medical Colleges affirms the value of diversity within the veterinary medical profession. The membership is committed to incorporating that belief into their actions by advocating the recruitment and retention of underrepresented persons as students and faculty and ultimately fostering their success in the profession of veterinary medicine. The Association believes that through these actions society and the profession will be well served.

Many schools have programs designed to facilitate entry into, and retention by, veterinary programs nationwide. These programs are directed at several levels, from high-school students to the student who has already been accepted by a veterinary college. Most of these programs will accept students from every state, regardless of the school(s) to which an individual might eventually apply or attend.

Following is an alphabetical list of schools by state and a short explanation of their programs:

## Auburn University College of Veterinary Medicine

*Program:* Summer Laboratory Experience Program

*Description:* students who have demonstrated an interest in the biological or health sciences spend 10 weeks working in the laboratory of a senior research scientist. Whenever possible, students will design and conduct an experiment and present the results to students and faculty during an exit seminar. Orientation sessions provide the student with the basics of laboratory safety and an introduction to sterile technique. An enrichment program provides information on career-related opportunities and cultural programs.

*Eligibility:* minority high-school students who have completed high-school chemistry and have an ACT score ≥ 25 or SAT composite score ≥ 1100.

*Contact:* Coordinator of Recruiting, College of Veterinary Medicine, Auburn University AL 36849-5519; telephone: (334) 844-2685; fax: (334) 844-2723.

*Sponsorship:* National Institutes of Health, National Center for Research Resources.

## University of California

*Program:* Summer Enrichment Program

*Description:* a 6-week summer residential program. The purpose of this program is to increase the academic preparedness of disadvantaged students through science-based learning skills development, clinical education, individual advising, and student development.

*Eligibility:* Educationally and/or economically disadvantaged. Must have completed at least one year of college with a minimum science GPA of 2.50 and demonstrated interest in veterinary medicine.

*Program dates:* July–August.

*Contact:* Office of the Dean, School of Veterinary Medicine, University of California, One Shields Avenue, Davis CA 95616; telephone: (530) 752-1383.

*Sponsorship:* School of Veterinary Medicine, University of California-Davis.

## Colorado State University

*Program:* Vet Prep

*Description:* a one-year academic program that serves as a bridge to the professional veterinary medical program for disadvantaged (cultural, social, economic) applicants who ranked high but were denied admission during the current admissions process. Limited to 7 students who upon successful completion are guaranteed admission to the veterinary program.

*Eligibility:* disadvantaged students.

*Contact:* College of Veterinary Medicine and Biomedical Sciences, W100 Anatomy, Colorado State University, Fort Collins CO 80523; telephone: (970) 491-7052.

*Sponsorship:* College of Veterinary Medicine and Biomedical Sciences, Colorado State University.

*Program:* Vet Start

*Description:* a 7-year undergraduate and professional program for students who come to Colorado State from high school or with fewer than 15 semester credits of college coursework. Undergraduate and professional program scholarships are provided, and admission to the professional veterinary medical program is guaranteed upon successful completion of the undergraduate requirements. Mentoring, support services, and summer jobs are also provided.

*Eligibility:* students who have a disadvantaged background (economic, cultural, or social) will be given special consideration. Students must be high-school graduates with fewer than 15 semester credits of college coursework.

15

Selection is competitive. There are 5 positions per year for incoming freshman undergraduate students.

*Program dates:* begins fall semester; applications available January 1; application deadline March 15.

*Contact:* College of Veterinary Medicine and Biomedical Sciences, W100 Anatomy, Colorado State University, Fort Collins CO 80523; telephone: (970) 491-7052.

*Sponsorship:* College of Veterinary Medicine and Biomedical Sciences, Colorado State University, and the U.S. Department of Agriculture.

## Cornell University

*Program:* State University of New York Graduate Underrepresented Minority Fellowships

*Description:* all matriculating underrepresented minorities are eligible (not restricted by state residency). Minority fellowships include a stipend.

*Contact:* Director of Financial Aid, College of Veterinary Medicine, S2-008 Schurman Hall, Cornell University, Ithaca NY 14853-6401; telephone (607) 253-3766.

*Program:* Regents Professional Opportunities Scholarships

*Description:* a financial assistance program for New York residents who are underrepresented minorities. Must agree to work in New York for a time after graduation.

*Contact:* Director of Financial Aid, College of Veterinary Medicine, S2-008 Schurman Hall, Cornell University, Ithaca NY 14853-6401; telephone (607) 253-3766.

## University of Illinois

*Program:* Multicultural Fellowhips

*Description:* to enhance the diversity of the student body and the profession, two $8,000 multicultural fellowships will be available to members of the incoming class. Fellowships are good for four years. Recipients must remain in good academic standing and work with the Office of Academic and Student Affairs with recruiting efforts.

## Michigan State University

*Program:* Vetward Bound Program

*Description:* Vetward Bound offers 3 levels of programming, each with its own eligibility requirements. The program provides a review of basic science content, research and/or clinical experience, preparation for the GRE and MCAT, veterinary experience, food and fiber animal experience, study strategy development, and field experiences. Placement in a specific level is determined by program staff and is based on educational background.

*Eligibility:* multicultural and/or educationally/economically disadvantaged first-year students through prematriculants into the professional degree program.

*Program dates:* June–July.

*Contact:* Vetward Bound Coordinator, College of Veterinary Medicine, A-136 East Fee Hall, Michigan State University, East Lansing MI 48824-1316; telephone: (517) 355-6521; e-mail: vetbound@cvm.msu.edu.

## Mississippi State University

*Program:* Board of Trustees of State Institutions of Higher Learning Veterinary Medicine Minority Loan/Scholarship Program

*Description:* a financial assistance program for Mississippi residents who are underrepresented minorities. Must agree to work in Mississippi for at least 3 years following graduation.

*Contact:* Director of Student Financial Aid, Mississippi Institutions of Higher Learning, 3825 Ridgewood Road, Jackson MS 39211-6453; telephone: (601) 982-6570.

## University of Missouri

*Program:* Gateway and Threshold to Veterinary Medicine

*Description:* 6-week summer programs which provide opportunities to gain experience with faculty researchers and clinicians in the field of veterinary medicine. Travel expenses, room, and board are provided. A stipend is also offered for miscellaneous expenses.

*Eligibility:* educationally or economically disadvantaged college sophomore, junior, and senior students.

*Program dates:* mid-June into July.

*Contact:* Associate Dean, College of Veterinary Medicine, University of Missouri, Columbia MO 65211.

## North Carolina State University

*Program:* Minority Presence Grants

*Description:* this annual program provides up to $4,000 annually to African-American North Carolina residents attending the College of Veterinary Medicine.

*Contact:* Student Services, College of Veterinary Medicine, (919) 513-6205, www.cvm.ncsu.edu.

*Program:* Native American Incentive Grant

*Description:* this annual program provides up to $4,900 annually to Native American North Carolina residents attending the College of Veterinary Medicine.

*Contact:* Student Services, College of Veterinary Medicine, (919) 513-6205, www.cvm.ncsu.edu.

## Ohio State University

*Program:* Young Scholars Program

*Description:* this summer program is offered to seventh- through eleventh-grade students from Ohio. It provides hands-on science activities, academic enrichment exercises, and career exploration opportunities.

*Eligibility:* disadvantaged students recommended by their faculty.

*Program dates:* June to August each summer.

*Sponsorship:* the State of Ohio and The Ohio State University.

*Program:* Summer Research Opportunity Program

*Description:* this program is designed to promote the migration of minority undergraduate students into graduate research educational programs by providing them with summer research experiences. The student is provided with his or her individualized research problem by a faculty mentor and expected to carry that research through to publication.

*Eligibility:* the student must have completed 2 years of college work and have achieved at least a 2.50 cumulative GPA. The student must be an under-represented minority or economically disadvantaged.

*Contact:* Graduate School, The Ohio State University, 230 North Oval Mall, Columbus OH 43210.

*Sponsorship:* the Big Ten Consortium for Institutional Studies.

## University of Tennessee

*Program:* Program for African-American High-School Students

*Description:* provides students with an opportunity to work with veterinarians in their hometowns for 8 weeks during the summer. During 2 weeks, students will be guests of the College of Veterinary Medicine on the campus of the University of Tennessee, Knoxville.

*Eligibility:* African-American juniors or seniors who are residents of Tennessee and enrolled in a Tennessee high school. Applicants must have an interest in veterinary medicine as a potential career. Preference will be given to seniors. Students receive an hourly wage for a 40-hour week.

*Program dates:* summer.

*Contact:* Associate Dean, University of Tennessee, College of Veterinary Medicine, P.O. Box 1071, Knoxville TN 37901-1071.

## Tuskegee University

*Program:* Health Careers Opportunity Program

*Description:* this 8-week preadmission activity is designed to facilitate the entry of "at risk" students and provide the skills necessary for successful transition to the professional school.

*Eligibility:* participation is targeted to minority and disadvantaged students who have completed at least 2 years of college and all preveterinary prerequisites. Participation is restricted to persons who have applied to the College of Veterinary Medicine, Nursing, and Allied Health and who have been selected by the Veterinary Admissions Committee to attend the program.

*Program dates:* summer before matriculation.

*Contact:* Assistant Dean, College of Veterinary Medicine, Nursing, and Allied Health, Tuskegee University, Tuskegee AL 36088.

*Sponsorship:* this program is sponsored by a grant from the U.S. Department of Health and Human Services.

*Program:* Veterinary Science Training, Education and Preparation Institutes for Minority Students (Vet-Step I and II)

*Description:* Consists of 2 one-week programs designed to encourage high-achieving minority students to consider veterinary medicine as a career choice. The program offers students progressive learning experiences in reading comprehension, note-taking, medical vocabulary, etc. Vet-Step II accepts high-school seniors and those students who have participated in Vet-Step I.

*Eligibility:* Vet-Step I accepts 25 students from grades 10 and 11; Vet-Step II accepts students from Vet-Step I and from grade 12. Minority high-school honor students interested in the biomedical sciences are eligible to apply.

*Program dates:* July.

*Contact:* Coordinator, Vet-Step Program, College of Veterinary Medicine, Nursing, and Allied Health, Tuskegee University, Tuskegee AL 36088.

*Sponsorship:* U.S. Department of Health and Human Services.

## Virginia-Maryland Regional College

*Program:* Minority Summer Research Program—Blacksburg

*Description:* a 10-week program providing opportunities to conduct scientific research; participate in clinical rotations within the veterinary teaching hospital; improve leadership, public speaking, and self-marketing skills; attend GRE preparatory classes; and learn about admission into graduate/ professional school.

*Contact:* Admissions Office at Blacksburg campus.

*Program:* Summer Research Apprenticeship Program—College Park

*Description:* a summer research program providing research experience to veterinary and preveterinary students from diverse backgrounds, including economic hardship and underrepresented racial/ethnic groups. Projects may include assisting in the planning, preparation, and data collection for controlled experiments, clinical trials, or epidemiological investigations; researching disease processes; and performing literature searches.

*Contact:* Admissions Office at College Park campus.

*Scholarship Opportunities:* a limited number of scholarships are available to assist minority DVM students.

## Washington State University

*Program:* Short-Term Research Training Program for Veterinary Students

*Description:* a 3-month summer program designed to promote interest in research by veterinary students. Emphasis is on a hands-on research project supervised by a faculty member with a research program. Stipends are provided.

*Eligibility:* Washington-Oregon-Idaho program veterinary students or ethnic minority veterinary students from other North American colleges of veterinary medicine.

*Program dates:* 3 months in the summer dependent upon the summer vacation of the College of Veterinary Medicine in which the veterinary student is enrolled.

*Contact:* Department of Veterinary Microbiology and Pathology, Washington State University, Pullman WA 99164-7040.

*Sponsorship:* The National Center for Research Resources.

**University of Wisconsin**

*Program:* Pre-College Enrollment Opportunity Program for Learning Excellence (PEOPLE)

*Description:* this program began in the summer of 1999 as a partnership between the Milwaukee Public Schools and the UW-Madison with a group of students who had just completed the ninth grade. New classes will be added each year, expanding to Madison area schools. The program is designed with a precollege track and a bridge program to undergraduate work and continues through a student's undergraduate career at University of Wisconsin-Madison. The main purposes are to promote academic preparation, increase enrollment in postsecondary institutions, and improve retention and graduation rates of minority students.

*Eligibility:* students of one or more of the following ethnic heritages: African American, American Indian, Asian American, Hispanic/Latino. Other eligibility factors include economic disadvantage and current enrollment in or commitment to a college preparatory curriculum track.

*Program dates:* June–July summer residential programs and year-round nonresidential programs.

*Contact:* Assistant Vice Chancellor, 117 Bascom Hall, University of Wisconsin-Madison, Madison, WI 53706; or Associate Director, University of Wisconsin-Madison Undergraduate Admissions, Armory and Gymnasium, 716 Langdon Street, Madison, WI 53706.

*Program:* University of Wisconsin-Madison NASA Sharp Plus Program

*Description:* an 8-week residential precollege program designed to increase the participation and success rates of students from minority groups that are historically underrepresented in mathematics and sciences. Students are matched with mentors (professors and research scientists) who are currently engaged in scientific research at the university or in an industrial setting.

*Eligibility:* rising high-school juniors or seniors who are U.S. citizens or nationals, at least 16 years of age, and have completed at least the tenth grade by the start of the program; have completed at least one semester of algebra and geometry and at least one year of biology, chemistry, or physics with a grade of B or better in each of these courses; speak and write English at a level that does not require significant assistance; and are committed to full participation throughout the 8-week program.

*Program dates:* June–August.

*Contact:* Assistant Vice Chancellor, Room 117 Bascom Hall, University of Wisconsin-Madison, Madison, WI 53706; or Program Coordinator, Uni-

versity of Wisconsin-Madison Medical School, 1140C Medical Science
Center, Madison, WI 53706

*Sponsorship:* Quality Education for Minorities and NASA.

*Scholarships:* the School of Veterinary Medicine has a scholarship and other
support funding available for preferred students. A portion of those funds
come from private donors earmarked specifically for underrepresented
groups and individuals who have experienced long-term disadvantages.

A professor of toxicology lectures in the poison plant garden at
the University of Illinois College of Veterinary Medicine. Photo
by Lil Morales, courtesy of the University of Illinois College of
Veterinary Medicine.

# Financial Aid Information

Financing your veterinary medical education requires careful planning, good money management skills, and a willingness to make short-term sacrifices to achieve long-range goals.

Many of you will apply for and receive some type of financial assistance during your undergraduate education. This will help you become somewhat familiar with the process, and to know that the rules and regulations governing programs can and do change periodically.

As a professional student, you will be entering a partnership with the financial aid office, which will require you to complete the appropriate financial aid forms accurately, meet required deadlines, and submit any additional information that may be requested. In return, the financial aid office will determine your aid eligibility and make awards based on the available programs. Your financial aid eligibility takes into account the cost of your education minus any other available resources. Amounts of assistance and the school policies for awarding assistance vary from one veterinary medical school to another and from year to year.

Any questions or concerns that you may have about this topic need to be directed to each of the appropriate financial aid offices to ensure that you receive accurate information and guidance.

# Financing Your Veterinary Medical Education

Your education is one of the biggest investments you will make in your lifetime, and one of your most important goals should be to maximize the return on all of your investments. To reach this goal, you must take an active role in managing your financial resources. You need to understand and implement good financial practices. To get you started, here are some good financial habits you should adopt:

- Do not use credit cards to extend your lifestyle. Deciding not to use credit cards except in emergencies is one of the most important decisions you can make, and one that will reduce your stress while you are pursuing your education.

- Budget your money just as carefully as you budget your time. Contact a financial aid administrator to help you set up a budget that will be easy to follow.

- Distinguish between wants and needs. Before you make any purchase, you should ask yourself, "Do I need this, or do I want it?"

- Be a well-informed borrower. If you have not previously taken an active role in understanding the differences between various student loan programs, now is the time to do it. You need to know these differences in order to avoid high-interest loans and to borrow wisely.

- Borrow the minimum amount necessary in order to maximize the return on your educational investment.

- Be thrifty. Live as cheaply as you can. Remember, you are a student. You'll enjoy a more comfortable lifestyle once you are a DVM.

- Pay any interest that accrues on student loans if you can afford to do so, rather than let the interest accrue and capitalize. Any amount you pay while you're a student will save you money once you enter repayment.

What is the most important piece of advice for making the most of your educational investment? Don't live the lifestyle of a DVM until you have completed your education. Get in the habit of being thrifty. If you live like a DVM while you are in school, you may have to live like a student when you are a DVM.

# Federal Loan Programs

|  | Subsidized Stafford Loan | Unsubsidized Stafford Loan |
|---|---|---|
| **Lender** | Financial or credit institution or eligible school | Financial or credit institution or eligible school |
| **Financial Need** | Yes | No |
| **Citizenship Requirement** | U.S. Citizen, U.S. National or U.S. Permanent Resident | U.S. Citizen, U.S. National or U.S. Permanent Resident |
| **Borrowing Limits** | $8,500/year; $65,500 aggregate undergraduate and graduate | Cost of attendance minus other aid; $189,125 aggregate undergraduate and graduate, less the Subsidized Stafford Loan Total |
| **Interest Rate** | Variable; capped at 8.25% | Variable; capped at 8.25% |
| **Interest Accrues School** | No | Yes |
| **Deferments** | No | Yes |
| **Grace Period** | No | Yes |

| Perkins Loan | Health Professions Student Loan | Loan for Disadvantaged Students |
|---|---|---|
| Veterinary Medicine Financial Aid Office | Veterinary Medicine Financial Aid Office | Veterinary Medicine Financial Aid Office |
| Yes | Yes | Yes |
| U.S. Citizen, U.S. National or U.S. Permanent Resident | U.S. Citizen, U.S. National or U.S. Permanent Resident | U.S. Citizen, U.S. National or U.S. Permanent Resident |
| $6,000/year; $40,000 aggregate undergraduate and graduate | Cost of attendance | Cost of attendance |
| 5% | 5% | 5% |
| No | No | No |
| No | No | No |
| No | No | No |

# Information about Standardized Tests

Most veterinary medical colleges require one or more standardized tests: the Medical College Admission Test (MCAT), Veterinary College Admission Test (VCAT), or Graduate Record Examination (GRE). For further information regarding test dates and registration procedures, contact the testing agencies listed below:

GRE
Graduate Record Examination
P.O. Box 6000
Princeton NJ 08541-6000
(609) 771-7670 (Princeton, N.J.)
also: (510) 654-1200 (Oakland, Calif.)
Individual School codes: see GRE booklet

MCAT
Medical College Admission Test
MCAT Program Office
P.O. Box 4056
Iowa City IA 52243
(319) 337-1357
VMCAS code 900

VCAT
The Psychological Corporation
Veterinary College Admission Test
555 Academic Court
San Antonio TX 78204
(210) 921-8794
(800) 622-3231
VMCAS code 44

TOEFL
Test of English as a Foreign Language
TOEFL/TSE Services
P.O. Box 6151
Princeton NJ 08541-6151
(609) 771-7100
VMCAS code 4936

# Veterinary Medical College Application Service (VMCAS)

The Veterinary Medical College Application Service has been established by the Association of American Veterinary Medical Colleges for applicants wishing to apply to colleges of veterinary medicine in the United States and Canada. VMCAS is a centralized application service that provides for the collection, processing, verification, and distribution of applicant data to the participating colleges for their use in the applicant selection process. *This service is a data-processing component of the admissions cycle only; it is in no way a part of the decision-making process, which is the prerogative of the admissions committees at the various colleges of veterinary medicine.*

Application deadlines, prerequisite courses, and other aspects of the selection process differ from college to college. Applicants must pay particular attention to the information and instructions included in the application packet for each of the participating colleges. Questions about the service may be directed to VMCAS, 1101 Vermont Avenue NW, Suite 411, Washington DC 20005-3521. Phone: (202) 682-0750; E-mail: VMCAS@aavmc.org; Web: www.aavmc.org/vmcas. (TTY) (202) 371-0899.

Fish health and aquaculture is an expanding field of study at some veterinary medical colleges. Photo courtesy of Atlantic Veterinary College, University of Prince Edward Island.

# Veterinary Medical Schools in the United States

## Auburn University

Office for Academic Affairs
College of Veterinary Medicine
217 Goodwin Student Center
Auburn University AL 36849-5536
Telephone: (334) 844-2685
E-mail: admiss@vetmed.auburn.edu
www.vetmed.auburn.edu

The College of Veterinary Medicine at Auburn University is located in south central Alabama on Interstate 85 between Montgomery and Atlanta. The university is known for its friendly small-campus atmosphere despite having more than 21,000 students.

Veterinary medicine began as a department at Auburn in 1892 and became a college in 1907. Today it is situated on 240 acres one mile from the main Auburn campus. In addition, the college has a 700-acre research farm five miles from its campus. The college is fully accredited by the American Veterinary Medical Association.

### Application Information

For specific application information (availability, deadlines, fees, and VMCAS participation), please refer to the contact information listed above.

*Residency implications:* priority is given to Alabama residents. Auburn contracts with Kentucky for 34 positions. Up to 10 nonresident students are accepted.

### Prerequisites for Admission

*Course requirements and semester hours*

|  |  |  |
|---|---|---|
|  | Written composition[#] | 6 |
| * | Literature[#] | 3 |
|  | Fine Arts[#] | 3 |
|  | Humanities/fine arts elective[#] | 6 |
| * | History[#] | 3 |
|  | Social/behavioral science electives[#] | 9 |

| | | |
|---|---|---|
| Mathematics — precalculus with trigonometry[#] | 3 |
| Principles of biology with lab | 4 |
| Animal biology with lab | 4 |
| Fundamentals of chemistry with lab | 8 |
| ** Organic chemistry with lab | 6 |
| ** Physics | 8 |
| Biochemistry | 3 |
| Science electives (jr. [300] level or above) | 6 |

*  Students must complete a 6-semester-hour sequence either in literature or in history.
** Organic chemistry and physics must have been taken within 6 calendar years.
#  These requirements will be waived if the student has a bachelor's degree.

*Required undergraduate GPA:* a minimum grade point average of at least 2.50 on a 4.00 scale is required, with the minimum acceptable grade for required courses being C-minus. Applicants not classified as Alabama residents or contract students must have a minimum 3.00 GPA on a 4.00 scale. The mean grade point average of the most recent entering class was 3.53.

*AP credit policy:* must appear on official college transcripts and be equivalent to the appropriate college-level coursework.

*Course completion deadline:* prerequisite courses must be completed by June 15 prior to matriculation.

*Standardized examinations:* Graduate Record Examination (GRE), general test, is required. The exam must have been taken within the previous 6 calendar years, and no later than October 1 of the year of application.

*Additional requirements and considerations*
    Animal/veterinary experience
    Recommendations (3 required)
        Academic advisor or faculty member
        Employer
        Veterinarian
    Extracurricular and community service activities
    Employment record
    Narrative statement of purpose
    Neatness of application
    Organic chemistry and physics courses must have been completed within
        the previous 6 calendar years

## Summary of Admission Procedure

*Timetable*
Application deadline: October 1
Date interviews are held: February–March
Date acceptances mailed: March
School begins: August

*Deposit* (to hold place in class): none required.

*Deferments:* not considered.

*Evaluation criteria*
The 3-part admission procedure includes an objective evaluation of academic credentials, a subjective review of personal credentials, and a personal interview by invitation.

*2000–2001 admissions summary*

|  | Number of Applicants | Number of New Entrants |
|---|---|---|
| Resident | 154 | 46 |
| Contract* | 100 | 34 |
| Nonresident | 601 | 10 |
| Total: | 855 | 90 |

## Expenses for the 2000-2001 Academic Year

*Tuition and fees*
| | |
|---|---|
| Resident | $6,500.00 |
| Nonresident | |
| Contract* | $6,500.00 |
| Other nonresident | $19,500.00 |

\* For further information, see the listing of contracting states and provinces.

# University of California

Office of the Dean — Student Programs
School of Veterinary Medicine
University of California
One Shields Avenue
Davis CA 95616
Telephone: (530) 752-1383
www.ucdavis.edu

The University of California, Davis (UCD) campus is adjacent to the city of Davis, which is 14 miles west of Sacramento, the state capital, and 72 miles northeast of San Francisco. Davis is known as the "city of bicycles." The community is closely tied to the university yet has developed its own recreational, cultural, and community outlets. Winter temperatures are generally mild and rarely fall below freezing. Summers are sunny, hot, and dry. Weather in the spring and fall is the most pleasant in the state. UCD is an outstanding research and training institution with approximately 24,500 undergraduate, graduate, and professional students enrolled in 4 colleges and professional schools (Veterinary Medicine, Medicine, Law, and Management). The educational buildings and research facilities are situated on over 5,200 acres at Davis and 10 off-campus field stations. UCD is the home of the Veterinary Medical Teaching Hospital, the California Regional Primate Research Center, the California Animal Health and Food Safety Laboratory System, the Veterinary Medical Teaching and Research Center, and the Center for Comparative Medicine. There are many innovative programs at UCD with many international students. The school is fully committed to recruiting students with diverse backgrounds.

## Application Information

For specific application information (availability, deadlines, fees, and VMCAS participation), please refer to the contact information listed above.

*Residency implications:* priority is given to California residents. California accepts no more than a total of 2 applicants from WICHE states (Alaska, Arizona, Hawaii, Montana, Nevada, New Mexico, North Dakota, Utah, and Wyoming), and California may accept a small number of uniquely qualified nonresident applicants.

## Prerequisites for Admission

*Course requirements and quarter hours*

| | |
|---|---|
| General chemistry (with laboratory) | 15 |
| Organic chemistry (with laboratory) | 6 |
| Biochemistry* (bioenergetics and metabolism) | 4 |
| Physics | 6 |
| Biology and zoology (1 laboratory requirement) | 10 |
| Systemic physiology* | 5 |
| Vertebrate embryology* | 4 |
| Genetics* | 4 |
| English composition and additional English | 12 |
| Humanities and social sciences | 12 |
| Statistics | 4 |

\* Upper-division courses equivalent to one semester or one quarter

Note: equivalent courses may vary in units and may also require other prerequisites.

*Required undergraduate GPA:* a minimum grade point average of 2.50 on a 4.00 scale is required for *both* the required sciences and cumulative college coursework. Applicants admitted in fall 2000 had a mean cumulative GPA of 3.45.

*AP credit policy:* must appear on official college transcripts.

*Course completion deadline:* all prerequisite courses must be completed by the time a student plans to enroll.

*Standardized examinations:* Graduate Record Examination (GRE), general test, is required. The most recent acceptable GRE test date for applicants entering fall 2002 is September 30, 2001. Date of oldest acceptable scores is October 1996. Average GRE scores for the class admitted in 2000 are verbal 595, quantitative 700, and analytical 724.

*Additional requirements and considerations*
Veterinary/animal experience
Letters of evaluation (3)
Personal statement of motivation/career goals
Accuracy and neatness of application
Interview/essay

## Summary of Admission Procedure

*Timetable*
    Application deadline: October 1
    Date interviews are held: February to mid-March
    Date acceptances mailed: by April 1
    School begins: early September

*Deposit (to hold place in class):* none required.

*Deferments:* not considered.

| Evaluation criteria | % weight |
|---|---|
| Grades | 28 |
| Test scores | 28 |
| Personal Statement/Essay/Animal and Veterinary Experience/References/Other | 24 |
| Interview | 20 |

*2000-2001 admissions summary*

| | Number of Applicants | Number of New Entrants |
|---|---|---|
| Resident | 499 | 116 |
| Contract* | 84 | 2 |
| Nonresident | 527 | 4 |
| Total: | 1,110 | 122 |

## Expenses for the 2000-2001 Academic Year

*Tuition and fees*
| | |
|---|---|
| Resident | $10,762.00 |
| Nonresident | $21,005.00 |
| Contract student* | $21,005.00 |

\* For further information, see the listing of contracting states and provinces.

## Dual-Degree Programs

Combined DVM-graduate degree programs are available.

# Colorado State University

Office of the Dean
College of Veterinary Medicine and Biomedical Sciences
Colorado State University
Fort Collins CO 80523-1601
Telephone: (970) 491-7052
E-mail: pvmadv@cvmbs.colostate.edu
www.cvmbs.colostate.edu

Colorado State University is located in Fort Collins, a city of about 109,000 in the eastern foothills of the Rocky Mountains about 60 miles north of Denver. Fort Collins has a pleasant climate and offers many cultural and recreational activities. Many of the state's ski areas lie within a short driving distance, making some of the best skiing in the world accessible. The nearby river canyons and mountain parks are beautiful scenic attractions and provide opportunities for hiking, fishing, photography, camping, and biking.

The College of Veterinary Medicine and Biomedical Sciences is composed of 5 major buildings, which house the departments of anatomy and neurobiology, microbiology, environmental health, pathology, physiology, and radiological health sciences. The Veterinary Teaching Hospital, one of the world's largest and best-equipped, houses the clinical sciences department. The hospital attracts a large caseload and offers students a wide variety of clinical experiences.

## Application Information

For specific application information (availability, deadlines, fees, and VMCAS participation), please refer to the contact information listed above.

*Residency implications:* positions are allocated as follows: Colorado 75, WICHE contracts 30–40 (Arizona, Hawaii, Montana, Nevada, New Mexico, North Dakota, Utah, Wyoming), and nonsponsored 10–20. WICHE students must be certified by their states. Nonsponsored students can be from any state or country.

## Prerequisites for Admission

*Course requirements and semester hours*

| | |
|---|---|
| Laboratory associated with a biology course | 1 |
| Genetics | 3 |
| Laboratory associated with a chemistry course | 1 |

| Biochemistry | 3 |
| Physics (with laboratory) | 4 |
| Statistics/biostatistics | 3 |
| English composition | 3 |
| Social sciences and humanities | 12 |
| Electives | 38 |

*Required undergraduate GPA:* the mean GPA for the 2000 matriculated class was 3.60 on a 4.00 scale.

*AP credit policy:* must appear on official college transcripts.

*Course completion deadline:* transcripts with final grades, including all required courses, must be received by July 15 prior to matriculation.

*Standardized examinations:* Graduate Record Examination (GRE), general test, is required and must be taken within the last five years prior to application. Scores must be received by October 1, 2001. Mean GRE scores for the 2000 matriculated class were verbal 511, quantitative 612, analytical 640.

*Additional requirements and considerations*
   Animal/veterinary/unique work experience
   Recommendations (3 preferred)
      Academic (academic advisor or college professor)
      Employer
      Veterinarian
   Essay
   Extracurricular and community service activities, leadership
   Quality of academic program (course load, challenging curriculum, honors)
   Contributions to diversity, extenuating circumstances

## Summary of Admission Procedure

*Timetable*
   Application deadline: October 1
   Date interviews are held: early February
   School begins: late August

*Deposit (to hold place in class):* none required.

*Deferments:* not considered.

*Evaluation criteria*
   Grades, quality of academic program
   GRE scores

Animal/veterinary/other work experience
Activities & achievements, community service
Essay
Letters of recommendation
Interview (Colorado only)

*2000–2001 admissions summary*

|  | Number of Applicants | Number of New Entrants |
|---|---|---|
| Sponsored | 297 | 75 |
| Sponsored (WICHE)* | 196 | 45 |
| Nonsponsored | 811 | 14 |
| Total: | 1,304 | 134 |

## Expenses for the 2000–2001 Academic Year

*Tuition and fees* (first-year students only)
| Sponsored | $9,100.00 |
|---|---|
| Nonsponsored | $30,000.00 |

\* For further information, see the listing of contracting states and provinces.

## Dual-Degree Programs

Combined DVM–graduate degree programs are available.

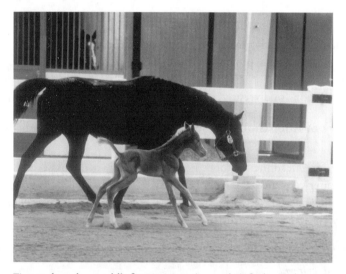

Firecracker, the world's first in-vitro (test tube) foal, was born at Colorado State University. Photo courtesy of College of Veterinary Medicine and Biomedical Sciences, Colorado State University.

# Cornell University

Office of DVM Admissions
College of Veterinary Medicine
S2-009 Schurman Hall
Cornell University
Ithaca, NY 14853-6401
Telephone: (607) 253-3700
E-mail: vet_admissions@cornell.edu
www.vet.cornell.edu

Cornell is located in Ithaca, a city of about 30,000 in the Finger Lakes region of upstate New York, a beautiful area of rolling hills, deep valleys, scenic gorges, and clear lakes. The university's 740-acre campus is bounded on two sides by gorges and waterfalls. Open countryside, state parks, and year-round opportunities for outdoor recreation, including excellent sailing, swimming, skiing, hiking, and other activities, are only minutes away.

Ithaca is one hour by air and a four-hour drive from New York City, and other major metropolitan areas are easily accessible. Direct commercial flights connect Ithaca with New York, Boston, Chicago, Pittsburgh, Washington, and other cities.

The tradition of academic excellence, the cultural vigor of a distinguished university, and the magnificent setting create a stimulating environment for graduate study. The curriculum differs from other programs in that it is interdisciplinary, tutorial-based learning early in the program and focuses on the student as the primary force in learning.

## Application Information

For specific application information (availability, deadlines, fees, and VMCAS participation), please refer to the contact information listed above.

*Residency implications:* approximately 60 positions for New York State residents. Cornell contracts with New Hampshire and New Jersey.

## Prerequisites for Admission

*Course requirements and semester hours*

| | |
|---|---|
| English composition* | 6 |
| Biology or zoology, full year with laboratory | 6 |
| Physics, full year with laboratory | 6 |

* Three credits may be satisfied by a course in public speaking.

| Inorganic (general) chemistry, full year with laboratory | 6 |
| Organic chemistry, full year with laboratory | 6 |
| Biochemistry | 4 |
| General microbiology, with laboratory | 3 |
| Electives | 53 |

All prerequisites must have a letter grade of C– or better.

*Required undergraduate GPA:* Cornell does not have a GPA requirement, but the grade range of those admitted tends to be 3.00–4.00. The median GPA for the class of 2004 was 3.60.

*AP credit policy:* not accepted for courses other than physics and inorganic chemistry.

*Course completion deadline:* all but 12 credits of the prerequisite coursework should be completed at the time of application, with at least one semester of any two-semester series underway. Any outstanding prerequisites must be completed by the end of the spring term prior to matriculation.

*Standardized examinations:* Graduate Record Examination (GRE), general test, is required. The most recent acceptable test date for applicants to the class of 2005 is the September 30, 2001 exam. The class of 2004 had a median score of 1350 (verbal 630 and quantitative 720). Test scores older than 5 years will not be accepted.

*Additional requirements and considerations*
   Animal/veterinary experience, knowledge, and motivation
   Recommendations/evaluations (3 required)
      Academic advisor
      Animal-experience employers
      Nonveterinary work-related experiences
   Essay
   Extracurricular and/or community service activities
   Demonstrated leadership skills
   Quality of academic program

## Summary of Admission Procedure

*Timetable*
   Application deadline: October 1
   Information sessions at the college: February–March
   Date acceptance mailed: February
   School begins: late August

*Deposit* (to hold place in class): $500.00.

*Deferments:* considered on an individual basis, but ordinarily granted only for illness or other problem beyond the voluntary control of the applicant.

*Evaluation criteria*

The admission procedure consists of 2 phases: an objective evaluation of academic credentials and a subjective review of the overall application.

|  | *% weight* |
|---|---|
| Grades | 30 |
| Test scores | 30 |
| Animal/veterinary experience | 20 |
| References, essay, quality of academic program, and nonacademic activities | 20 |

*2000-2001 admissions summary*

|  | *Number of Applicants* | *Number of New Entrants* |
|---|---|---|
| Resident | 274 | 50 |
| Contract* | 80 | 4 |
| Nonresident | 898 | 26 |
| Total: | 1,252 | 80 |

**Expenses for the 2000-2001 Academic Year**

*Tuition and fees*

| Resident | $15,400.00 |
|---|---|
| Nonresident | |
| Contract student* | $15,400.00 |
| Other nonresident | $21,100.00 |

\* For further information, see the listing of contracting states and provinces.

**Dual-Degree Programs**

Combined DVM-graduate degree programs are available.

**Early Admission Program**

The Leadership Training Program targets gifted first-year veterinary medical students who are potential leaders in the profession. The major objective of the program is to acquaint students with veterinary medical career opportunities in academic institutions, government, and industry. The program also encourages networking among the participants. Fellowships are available. For further information, contact: Graduate Education Coordinator, Schurman Hall, Cornell University, Ithaca, NY 14853; telephone (607) 253-3720.

# University of Florida

Admissions Office
College of Veterinary Medicine
P.O. Box 100125
University of Florida
Gainesville FL 32610-0125
Telephone: (352) 392-4700, ext. 5300
E-mail: henryt@mail.vetmed.ufl.edu
www.vetmed.ufl.edu

The University of Florida is located in Gainesville, a college town of approximately 100,000 in north central Florida, midway between the Gulf of Mexico and the Atlantic Ocean. Changes in season are marked, but winters are mild and permit year-round participation in outdoor activities.

The university accommodates about 40,000+ students with programs in almost all disciplines. The College of Veterinary Medicine is a component of the Institute of Food and Agriculture Sciences (which also includes Agriculture and Forest Resources and Conservation). It is also one of 6 colleges affiliated with the Health Science Center (the other 5 are Dentistry, Health-related Professions, Medicine, Nursing, and Pharmacy).

The veterinary curriculum is a 9-semester program consisting of core curriculum and elective experiences. The core provides the body of knowledge and skills common to all veterinarians. The first 4 semesters concentrate primarily on basic medical sciences. Students are additionally introduced to physical diagnosis, radiology, and clinical problems during these years. The core also includes experience in each of the clinical areas. Elective areas of concentration permit students to investigate further the aspects of both basic and clinical sciences most relevant to their interests.

## Application Information

For specific application information (availability, deadlines, fees, and VMCAS participation), please refer to the contact information listed above.

*Residency implications:* priority is given to Florida residents, and Florida has no contractual agreements. Nonresidents are considered in very limited numbers (not more than 15% of any entering class).

## Prerequisites for Admission

*Course requirements and semester hours*

| | |
|---|---|
| Biology (general, genetics, microbiology) | 15 |
| Chemistry (inorganic, organic, biochemistry) | 19 |
| Physics | 8 |
| Mathematics (calculus, statistics) | 6 |
| Animal Science (introduction to animal science, animal nutrition) | 6 |
| Humanities | 9 |
| Social sciences | 6 |
| English (2 courses in English composition) | 6 |
| Electives | at least 5 |

*Required undergraduate GPA:* a minimum GPA of 2.75 on a 4.00 scale. The class of 2004 had an overall mean science prerequisite GPA of 3.58.

*AP credit policy:* must appear on official college transcripts and be equivalent to the appropriate college-level coursework.

*Course completion deadline:* prerequisite courses must be completed by the end of the spring term prior to admission.

*Standardized examinations:* Graduate Record Examination (GRE) is required. October 2001 is the most recent acceptable test date for applicants to the class of 2005. Mean score for the class of 2004 was 1197.

*Additional requirements and considerations*

Animal/veterinary experience
Recommendations/evaluations (3 required)
    Personal
    Veterinarian
    Academic advisor
Honors and awards received
Extracurricular activities
Essay

## Summary of Admission Procedure

*Timetable*
   Application deadline: October 1
   Date interviews are held: March
   Date acceptances mailed: April 1
   School begins: mid-August

*Deposit* (to hold place in class): none required.

*Deferments:* considered on an individual basis.

*Evaluation criteria*
The admission procedure consists of 3 parts: each applicant's file is reviewed; selected applicants are each interviewed for about 20 minutes by 3 faculty members; final selection of new class takes place.

*2000-2001 admissions summary*

|  | | *Number of Applicants* | *Number of New Entrants* |
|---|---|---|---|
| Resident | | 289 | 74 |
| Contract | | N/A | N/A |
| Nonresident | | 613 | 5 |
| | Total: | 902 | 79 |

## Expenses for the 2000-2001 Academic Year

*Tuition and fees*
   Resident                        $8,631.00
   Nonresident                     $22,846.00

# University of Georgia

Office for Academic Affairs
College of Veterinary Medicine
The University of Georgia
Athens GA 30602-7372
Telephone: (706) 542-5728
E-mail: ywilson@calc.vet.uga.edu
www.vet.uga.edu

The University of Georgia is located in Athens-Clarke County, with a population of 86,000. Georgia's "Classic City" is a prospering community that reflects the charm of the Old South while growing in culture and industry. Athens is just over an hour away from the north Georgia mountains and the metropolitan area of Atlanta, and just over 5 hours away from the Atlantic coast.

In 1785, Georgia became the first state to grant a charter for a state-supported university. In 1801 the first students came to the newly formed frontier town of Athens. The University of Georgia has grown into an institution with 13 schools and colleges and more than 2,700 faculty members and 30,000 students.

## Application Information

For specific application information (availability, deadlines, fees, and VMCAS participation), please refer to the contact information listed above.

*Residency implications:* Georgia retains up to 25 positions for contract students. Contracts are with Delaware (maximum 2), South Carolina (maximum 17), and West Virginia (maximum 6). The balance of those admitted are residents of Georgia or nonresident, noncontract applicants.

## Prerequisites for Admission

*Course requirements and semester hours*

| | |
|---|---|
| English | 6 |
| Humanities and social studies | 14 |
| General biology | 8 |
| Advanced biological science | 8 |
| Chemistry | |
|     Inorganic | 8 |
|     Organic | 8 |
| Physics | 8 |
| Biochemistry | 3 |

*Required undergraduate GPA:* cumulative GPA of 3.00 or greater on a 4.00 scale *or* a combined score on the GRE verbal and quantitative sections of 1200 or greater.

*AP credit policy:* must appear on official college transcripts and be equivalent to the appropriate college-level coursework.

*Course completion deadline:* prerequisite courses must be completed by the end of the spring term preceding entry.

*Standardized examinations:* Graduate Record Examination (GRE), general test, and the biology subject test must be completed within the 5 years immediately preceding the deadline for receipt of applications (October 1). Test scores must be received by February 1 after the October 1 application deadline.

*Additional requirements and considerations*
    Animal experience
    Background for veterinary medicine
    Recommendations/evaluations (3 required)
        Academic advisor/faculty member (required for graduate students)
        Employer
        Veterinarian
    Essay

## Summary of Admission Procedure

*Timetable*
    Application deadline: October 1
    Date acceptances mailed: late March
    School begins: late August

*Deposit* (to hold place in class): $100.00; $500.00 for nonresident, noncontract students.

*Deferments:* one-year deferments considered for reasons such as completing a degree or for health problems.

*Evaluation criteria*
The admissions procedure includes a file evaluation. There are no interviews.

Academic performance
Standardized test scores
Animal/veterinary experience
References
Employment history
Narrative statement
Extracurricular activities

*2000–2001 admissions summary*

|  | Number of Applicants | Number Accepted |
|---|---|---|
| Resident | 191 | 61 |
| Contract* | 96 | 21 |
| Nonresident | 520 | 4 |
| Total: | 807 | 86 |

## Expenses for the 2000-2001 Academic Year

*Tuition and fees* (approximate)

| | |
|---|---|
| Resident | $6,834.00 |
| Nonresident | |
|   Contract* | $6,834.00 |
|   Nonresident | $19,109.00 |

\* For further information, see the listing of contracting states and provinces.

# University of Illinois

Office of Academic and Student Affairs
College of Veterinary Medicine
University of Illinois at Urbana-Champaign
2271G Veterinary Medicine Basic Sciences Bldg.
2001 South Lincoln Avenue
Urbana IL 61802
Telephone: (217) 333-1192
E-mail: admissions@cvm.uiuc.edu
www.cvm.uiuc.edu

The University of Illinois is in Urbana-Champaign, a community of about 100,000 people located 140 miles south of Chicago. It is served by 4 airlines, 3 interstate highways, bus, and rail. The twin cities and university make a pleasant community with easy access to all areas and facilities. The university has about 35,000 students and more than 11,000 faculty and staff members. It is known for its high-quality academic programs and its exceptional resources and facilities. The university library has the largest collection of any public university and ranks third among all U.S. academic libraries. The university also has outstanding cultural and sports facilities and activities.

The College of Veterinary Medicine is located at the south edge of the campus in a large physical plant built in phases since 1971. In addition to approximately 380 students, the college has about 100 graduate students plus a full complement of residents and interns. There are more than 100 full-time faculty with research interests in a variety of biomedical sciences and clinical areas. This research activity allows a variety of interactions and employment for students. The college also offers students a stimulating core-elective curriculum to prepare for a career in almost any area of the profession.

## Application Information

For specific application information (availability, deadlines, fees, and VMCAS participation), please refer to the contact information listed above.

*Residency implications:* priority is given to approximately 80 Illinois residents; approximately 20 nonresident positions.

## Prerequisites for Admission

The academic requirements for application to the College of Veterinary Medicine can be met through one of two pathways: Plan A or Plan B. Those considering a career in veterinary medicine should have a good foundation in biological sciences and chemistry, including *biochemistry,* and should consider the specific courses listed in Plan A as a minimum knowledge base for success in the curriculum. In addition, a course or courses concerning livestock production and animal ethology are highly desirable for all students. Those seeking a career in veterinary medicine related to agriculture should consider additional background in nutrition, livestock management, and the economics of production by working toward a degree in animal science prior to admission to veterinary school.

Plan A

BS or BA degree in any major field of study from an accredited college or university including the following courses (equivalent in content to those required for students majoring in biological sciences):
  a. 8 semester hours of biological sciences with laboratories
  b. 16 semester hours of chemical sciences, including organic and biochemistry, with laboratories in inorganic and organic chemistry
  c. 8 semester hours of physics with laboratories

Plan B

Those applying without a bachelor's degree are required to present at least 60 semester hours from an accredited college or university, including 40 hours of science courses. The minimum course requirements under Plan B are:
  a. 8 semester hours of biological sciences with laboratories
  b. 16 semester hours of chemical sciences, including organic and biochemistry, with laboratories in inorganic and organic chemistry
  c. 8 semester hours of physics with laboratories
  d. 3 semester hours of English composition and an additional 3 hours of English composition and/or speech
  e. 12 semester hours of humanities and social sciences
  f. 10 semester hours of junior/senior-level courses in addition to the requirements listed above

*Required undergraduate GPA:* a minimum cumulative GPA of 2.75 and a minimum science GPA of 2.75 on a 4.00 scale are required. The mean cumulative GPA for students invited to interview in 2000 was 3.67, mean science GPA was 3.62, and mean GRE score was 72 (percentile).

*AP credit policy:* not available.

*Standardized examinations:* Graduate Record Examination (GRE), general test, is required. Test must be taken by September 30 of the year of application, and scores may be no older than two years.

*Additional requirements and considerations*
　　Animal veterinary knowledge, motivation, and experience
　　Recommendations/evaluations
　　　　Animal- and veterinary-experience employer
　　　　Academic advisor
　　Evidence of leadership, initiative, and responsibility
　　Rigor of academic preparation

## Summary of Admission Procedure

*Timetable*
　　Application deadline: October 1
　　Informational program and required interviews: early March
　　Date acceptances mailed: mid-March
　　School begins: late August

*Deposit* (to hold place in class): none required.

*Deferments:* not considered.

*Evaluation criteria*
A 2-part admission procedure is used. A file evaluation, stressing academic achievement and personal qualities, is followed by a personal interview.

|  | % weight |
|---|---|
| Test scores | 20 |
| Science GPA | 25 |
| Cumulative GPA | 15 |
| Subjective points: | 30 |
| academic rigor, veterinary experience, animal experience, evidence of leadership ability, and letters of evaluation. | |
| Interview | 10 |

*2000–2001 admissions summary*

|  | Number of Applicants | Number of New Entrants |
|---|---|---|
| Resident | 248 | 83 |
| Nonresident | 822 | 21 |
| Total: | 1,070 | 104 |

## Expenses for the 2000-2001 Academic Year

*Tuition and fees*
| | |
|---|---|
| Resident | $10,090.00 |
| Nonresident | $24,872.00 |

## Dual-Degree Programs

Combined DVM–graduate degree programs are available.

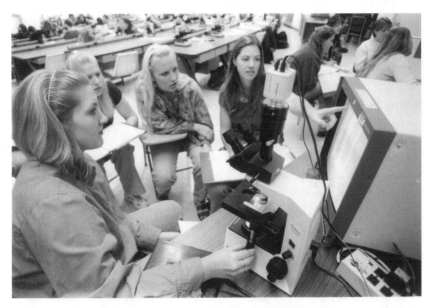

First-year veterinary students at the University of Illinois use a projection microscope to discuss histology slides. Photo by Don Hamerman, courtesy of the University of Illinois College of Veterinary Medicine.

# Iowa State University

Office of Admissions
College of Veterinary Medicine
2524 Veterinary Medicine
Iowa State University
Ames IA 50011-1250
Telephone: (515) 294-1242
Toll free outside Iowa: (800) 262-3810
E-mail: cvm_admissions@iastate.edu
www.vetmed.iastate.edu

The Iowa State University College of Veterinary Medicine is located in the heart of one of the world's most intensive livestock-producing areas, which provides diverse food-animal clinical and diagnostic cases. A nearby metropolitan area and a regionally recognized referral veterinary hospital provide experience in companion-animal medicine and surgery. A racetrack is located near the college and provides an increasing number of challenging equine patients.

A strong basic science education during the first 2 years prepares veterinary students for a wide range of clinical experiences during the last 2 years. The College of Veterinary Medicine provides education in a wide variety of animal species and disciplines and allows fourth-year students to spend time with private practitioners, other colleges, research facilities, and in other educational experiences. Opportunities for research exist in the outstanding research programs in neurobiology, immunobiology, infectious diseases, and numerous other areas, and the nearby National Animal Disease Center and the National Veterinary Services Laboratories provide additional opportunities. The world's premier State Diagnostic Laboratory is part of the college and provides students with experience that is unmatched by any other veterinary college in the world. Graduates are highly sought after and can typically choose among 5 or 6 job offers. A career development and placement service is also provided.

## Application Information

For specific application information (availability, deadlines, fees, and VMCAS participation), please refer to the contact information listed above.

*Residency implications:* priority is given to Iowa residents for approximately 60 positions. Iowa contracts on a year-to-year basis with New Jersey, North Dakota, and South Dakota. Remaining positions are available for residents of noncontract states or international students.

## Prerequisites for Admission*

*Course requirements and semester hours*

| | |
|---|---|
| English composition (includes business and/or technical writing | 6 |
| General chemistry (with laboratory) | 8 |
| Organic chemistry (with laboratory) | 7 |
| Biochemistry | 3 |
| Physics (with laboratory) | 8 |
| Biology (with laboratory) | 8 |
| Genetics | 3 |
| Mammalian anatomy and/or physiology | 3 |
| Speech (public speaking) | 3 |
| Arts, humanities, or social sciences | 9 |
| Electives | 8 |

\* All required science courses must have been completed within the past 8 years.

*Required undergraduate GPA:* the minimum GPA required by Iowa State University is 2.50 on a 4.00 scale. The most recent entering class had a mean GPA of 3.57 with a range of 3.04 to 4.00.

*AP credit policy:* must be documented by original scores submitted to the university, and must meet the university's minimum requirement in the appropriate subject area. Credits accepted only for the arts, humanities, and social sciences.

*Course completion deadline:* prerequisite courses must be completed by the end of the spring term prior to matriculation with a grade of C or better. Pass-not pass grades are not acceptable. Students wishing to matriculate in fall 2003 must complete all science requirements by the end of the fall term of the year the applicant applies.

*Standardized examinations:* Graduate Record Examination (GRE), general test, is required.

*Additional requirements and considerations*
Recommendations (3 required). Academic advisors, veterinarians, and employers are suggested.

## Summary of Admission Procedure

*Timetable*
    Application deadline: October 1
    Date acceptances mailed: March 15
    School begins: late August

*Deposit* (to hold place in class): $250.00

*Deferments:* not considered.

*Evaluation criteria*
The admission procedure consists of a review of each candidate's application and qualifications:

1. Academic factors include grades, test scores, and degrees earned.
2. Nonacademic factors include personal statement, experience, recommendations, and personal development activities.

*2000–2001 admissions summary*

|  | Number of Applicants | Number of New Entrants |
|---|---|---|
| Resident | 134 | 61 |
| Contract* | 70 | 16 |
| Nonresident | 616 | 23 |
| Total: | 820 | 100 |

## Expenses for the 2000–2001 Academic Year

*Tuition and fees*
    Resident                  $6,630.00
    Nonresident
        Contract*         varies by contract
        Other nonresident    $18,074.00

\* For further information, see the listing of contracting states and provinces.

## Dual-Degree Programs

Combined DVM–graduate degree programs are available.

# Kansas State University

Office of Admissions
College of Veterinary Medicine
101 Trotter Hall
1700 Denison Avenue
Kansas State University
Manhattan KS 66506-5601
Telephone: (785) 532-4335
Fax: (785) 532-4850
E-mail: admit@vet.ksu.edu
www.vet.ksu.edu

Kansas State University in Manhattan, Kansas, is located 125 miles west of Kansas City near Interstate 70. With a population of about 60,000 including KSU, Manhattan is in an area surrounded by many historical points of interest in a rich agricultural area of north central Kansas. Recreational activities abound in Manhattan and the surrounding area with fishing, boating, camping, and hunting among the favorites. Sporting events, theater, concerts, and excellent parks contribute to the many activities available. Kansans enjoy the 4 seasons, each of which brings its own special activities and events.

Kansas State University is on a beautiful 664-acre campus. The College of Veterinary Medicine opened in 1905. It is located on 80 acres just north of the main campus in 3 connected buildings.

## Application Information

For specific application information (availability, deadlines, fees, and VMCAS participation), please refer to the contact information listed above.

*Residency implications:* priority is given to Kansas residents; to be eligible to be in the Kansas pool of applicants, the applicant must be a Kansas resident for tuition purposes at the time of application. Kansas contracts with Nebraska. Kansas accepts about 25 nonresident, noncontract students per year.

## Prerequisites for Admission

*Course Requirements and Semester Hours*

| | |
|---|---|
| Expository writing I and II | 6 |
| Public speaking | 2 |
| Chemistry I and II | 8 |
| General organic chemistry, with laboratory | 5 |

| General biochemistry, with laboratory | 5 |
| Physics I and II | 8 |
| Principles of biology or general zoology | 4 |
| Mammalian embryology, with laboratory, or developmental biology * | 4 |
| Microbiology, with laboratory | 4 |
| Animal genetics or general genetics | 3 |
| Social sciences and /or humanities | 12 |
| Electives | 9 |

\* If a course in embryology or developmental biology is not offered at the school you are attending, please contact the office of the Associate Dean.

All science courses must have been taken within six years of the date of enrollment in the professional program.

*Required undergraduate GPA:* the required GPA is a 2.80 on a 4.00 scale in both the prerequisite courses and the last 45 semester hours of undergraduate work. The most recent entering class had a mean prerequisite science GPA of 3.43.

*AP credit policy:* must appear on official college transcripts and be equivalent to the appropriate college-level coursework.

*Course completion deadline:* prerequisite courses must be completed by the end of the spring term of the year in which admission is sought.

*Standardized examinations:* Graduate Record Examination (GRE), general test, is required by October 1. Nonresident, noncontract applicants having combined scores of less than 1800 are not likely to be interviewed.

*Additional requirements and considerations*
    Animal/veterinary work experience and knowledge
    Employment record
    3 evaluations required by nonfamily members, one a veterinarian. Other suggested references include academic or preprofessional advisor, professor, or other professional.

## Summary of Admission Procedure

*Timetable*
Application deadline: October 1
Date interviews are held:
    Kansas residents: late December
    Nebraska residents: early February
    Nonresident: early January
Date acceptances mailed: within one month after interview
School begins: mid-August

*Deposit* (to hold place in class): $100.00 for Kansas and contract state residents, $250.00 for nonresident students.

*Deferments:* may be granted by Admissions Committee for extraordinary circumstances.

*Evaluation criteria*
A 4-part admission procedure is used, including evaluation of science grades, evaluation of all 3 GRE scores, assessment of the application and narrative, and a personal interview.

| | |
|---|---|
| Prerequisite science GPA | 30% |
| Test scores | 40% |
| Interview score including: | 30% |
|     References | |
|     Animal/veterinary experience | |
|     Leadership in college and community | |
|     Autobiographical essay | |

*2000–2001 admissions summary*

| | Number of Applicants | Number of New Entrants |
|---|---|---|
| Resident | 106 | 52 |
| Contract* | 40 | 22 |
| Nonresident | 413 | 26 |
| Total: | 559 | 100 |

\* For further information, see the listing of contracting states and provinces.

**Expenses for the 2000-2001 Academic Year**

*Tuition and fees* (subject to change)

| | |
|---|---|
| Resident | $6,880.00 |
| Nonresident | |
| Contract* | $6,880.00 |
| Other nonresident | $23,680.00 |

\* For further information, see the listing of contracting states and provinces.

**Dual-Degree Programs**

Combined DVM-graduate degree programs are available.

**Early Admission Program**

The Veterinary Scholars Early Admission Program is designed for those students having a genuine desire to enter the veterinary profession who attend Kansas State University with an ACT score of 29 or greater or a comparable composite SAT score and who complete a successful interview during the fall semester of their freshman undergraduate year.

# Louisiana State University

Office of Veterinary Student and Academic Affairs
School of Veterinary Medicine
Louisiana State University
Baton Rouge LA 70803
Telephone: (225) 578-9537
Fax: (225) 578-9546
E-mail: cmiceli@mail.vetmed.lsu.edu
www.vetmed.lsu.edu

The Louisiana State University campus is located in Baton Rouge, which has a population of more than 500,000 and is a major industrial city, a thriving port, and the state's capital. Since it is located on the Mississippi River, Baton Rouge was a target for domination by Spanish, French, and English settlers. The city bears the influence of all 3 cultures and offers a range of choices in everything from food to architectural design. Geographically, Baton Rouge is the center of south Louisiana's main cultural and recreational attractions. Equally distant from New Orleans and the fabled Cajun bayou country, there is an abundance of cultural and outdoor recreational activities. South Louisiana has a balmy climate that encourages lush vegetation and comfortable temperatures year round.

The campus encompasses more than 2,000 acres in the southern part of Baton Rouge and is bordered on the west by the Mississippi River. The Veterinary Medicine Building, occupied in 1978, houses the academic departments, the veterinary library, and the Veterinary Teaching Hospital and clinics. The school is fully accredited by the American Veterinary Medical Association.

## Application Information

For specific application information (availability, deadlines, fees, and VMCAS participation), please refer to the contact information listed above.

*Residency implications:* Louisiana contracts with Arkansas (9). Louisiana accepts up to 15 highly qualified nonresident applicants.

## Prerequisites for Admission

*Course requirements and semester hours*

| | |
|---|---|
| Biology | 8 |
| Microbiology | 4 |
| Physics | 6 |
| General chemistry | 8 |
| Organic chemistry | 3 |
| Biochemistry | 3 |
| English composition | 6 |
| Speech communication | 3 |
| Mathematics | 5 |
| Electives | 20 |

*Required undergraduate GPA:* the minimum acceptable GPA for required coursework is 2.50 on a 4.00 scale. The mean GPA of the most recent entering class at the time of acceptance was 3.55.

*AP credit policy:* must appear on official college transcripts and be equivalent to the appropriate college-level coursework.

*Course completion deadline:* prerequisite courses must be completed by the end of the spring term preceding matriculation.

*Standardized examinations:* Medical College Admission Test or Graduate Record Examination, general test, is required. The most recent acceptable test date is early fall of the year of application. The average GRE combined verbal and quantitative score was 1121 for the class of 2004.

*Additional requirements and considerations*
   Animal/veterinary work experience
   Motivation, maturity
   Demonstrated communication skills
   Breadth of interests

## Summary of Admission Procedure

*Timetable*
   Application deadline: October 1
   Date interviews are held: early March
   Date acceptances mailed: late March
   School begins: late August

*Deposit* (to hold place in class): $500.00 for nonresidents.

*Deferments:* considered.

*Evaluation criteria*

The approximate components of the evaluation scoring are:

*Objective evaluation:*

| | |
|---|---|
| GPA required courses | 32% |
| GPA last 45 hours | 20% |
| Test scores | 18% |

*Subjective evaluation:*

| | |
|---|---|
| Animal/veterinary experience, references (3 required, one by a veterinarian), essay | 16% |
| Personal interview | 10% |
| Committee evaluation | 4% |

*2000-2001 admissions summary*

| | | *Number of Applicants* | *Number of New Entrants* |
|---|---|---|---|
| Resident | | 209 | 66 |
| Contract* | | 67 | 9 |
| Nonresident | | 868 | 5 |
| | Total: | 1,144 | 80 |

## Expenses for the 2000-2001 Academic Year

*Tuition and fees* (estimated)

| | |
|---|---|
| Resident | $6,734.00 |
| Nonresident | |
| Contract* | $6,734.00 |
| Other nonresident | $19,484.00 |

\* Further information, see the listing of contracting states and provinces.

# Michigan State University

Office of Admissions
College of Veterinary Medicine
A-126 East Fee Hall
Michigan State University
East Lansing MI 48824-1316
Telephone: (517) 353-9793; fax: (517) 432-2391; helpline: (800) 496-4678
E-mail: admiss@cvm.msu.edu
www.cvm.msu.edu

Michigan State University's campus is bordered by the city of East Lansing, which offers sidewalk cafes, restaurants, shops, and convenient mass transit. The campus is traversed by the Red Cedar River and has many miles of bike paths and walkways. This park-like setting provides an ideal venue in which MSU's 41,000 students may enjoy outdoor concerts and plays, canoeing, and cross-country skiing. North of the river is the older part of campus. The ivy-covered buildings, some built before the Civil War and listed on the National Register of Historic Places, house 5 colleges, the student union, and 10 residence halls. South of the river are more recent additions to the campus, such as the Wharton Center for Performing Arts, the Jack Breslin Student Events Center, and several intramural sports facilities.

The college is a national leader in state-of-the-art technology and facilities. A lecture hall is equipped with a computer at each of the 116 work stations. These computers are part of a network that links all parts of the Veterinary Medical Center and allows instructors to receive immediate feedback on how well students understand the lecture material. The Veterinary Teaching Hospital has one of the largest caseloads in the country. Outstanding faculty are involved in teaching veterinary students, providing patient treatment and diagnostic services, and conducting veterinary research.

## Application Information

For specific application information (availability, deadlines, fees, and VMCAS participation), please refer to the contact information listed above.

*Residency implications:* priority given to Michigan residents. Admission of nonresident and international applicants is limited. Michigan State University has no contractual agreements.

## Prerequisites for Admission

*Course requirements and semester hours*
General education
    English composition     3
    Social and behavioral sciences     6
    Humanities     6
Mathematics and biological and physical sciences
    General inorganic chemistry (with laboratory)     3-5
    Organic chemistry (with laboratory)     6-8
    Biochemistry*     4
    General biology (with laboratory)     6-9
    College algebra and trigonometry     3-5
    College physics (with laboratory)     8

\*   This should be an upper-division course in general biochemistry.

*Required undergraduate GPA:* none; the mean cumulative GPA for the last entering class (fall 2000) was 3.61 on a 4.00 scale.

*AP credit policy:* not available.

*Course completion deadline:* prerequisite courses must be completed by the end of the summer session prior to matriculation.

*Standardized examinations:* Medical College Admission Test (MCAT) or the Graduate Record Examination (GRE), general test, is required no later than October. For applicants to the class of 2006, the most recent acceptable MCAT test scores are those of the August 2001 exam. The average MCAT scores for the class entering in 2000 were: verbal 7.94, physical sciences 9.00, and biological sciences 8.50. For applicants to the class of 2006, the most recent acceptable GRE test scores are those of the September 30, 2001 exam. For the class entering in 2000, average GRE scores were: verbal 486, quantitative 611, and analytical 627. The Test of English as a Foreign Language (TOEFL) is required for applicants whose primary language is not English.

*Additional requirements and considerations*
    Extracurricular and/or community service activities
    Veterinary-related experience
    Evaluations
        Veterinarian
        Applicant's choice (2)
        Academic advisor (required for graduate students)

## Summary of Admission Procedure

*Timetable*
    Application deadline: October 1
    Date interviews are held: January, February, and March
    Date acceptances mailed: early April
    School begins: late August

*Deposit (to hold place in class):* $250.00 for residents; $500.00 for nonresidents.

*Deferments:* are rare.

*Evaluation criteria*
The 2-phase admission process consists of an academic review and a non-academic review, including an interview and a pre-interview extemporaneous composition.

*2000–2001 admissions summary*

|  | Number of Applicants | Number of New Entrants |
|---|---|---|
| Resident | 202 | 80 |
| Nonresident | 1,051 | 24 |
| Total: | 1,253 | 104 |

## Expenses for the 2000-2001 Academic Year

*Tuition and fees*
| | |
|---|---|
| Resident | $11,490.00 |
| Nonresident | $23,694.00 |

## Early Admission Program

The Veterinary Scholars Admission Program has been established by the College of Veterinary Medicine in cooperation with the Honors College at Michigan State. This program provides an admission opportunity for students who wish to complete a bachelor's degree consisting of advanced, intellectually challenging, and scholarly studies in concert with their entry to the four-year professional veterinary medical degree program. Enrollment at MSU and membership in the Honors College are required to be eligible for this option. Further information may be obtained from the Pre-veterinary Advising Center at the address indicated on page 64. For information on Honors College membership, contact: Honors College, 103 Eustace Hall, Michigan State University, East Lansing, MI 48824; telephone (517) 355-2326; or e-mail: honors@pilot.msu.edu

# University of Minnesota

Office of Student Affairs and Admissions
College of Veterinary Medicine
460 Veterinary Teaching Hospital
1365 Gortner Avenue
University of Minnesota
St. Paul MN 55108
Telephone: (612) 624-4747
E-mail: bjork010etc.umn.edu
www.cvm.umn.edu

The University of Minnesota's College of Veterinary Medicine is located on the 540-acre St. Paul campus. Students enjoy a small-campus atmosphere as well as the academic, cultural, social, and recreational opportunities of a major university and large metropolitan area. Cultural life includes world-renowned institutions and a rich local mix of theater, music, and arts organizations. The Twin Cities also house the state capital and the headquarters of many diverse major corporations. Minneapolis and St. Paul consistently rank near the top on quality-of-life and residential satisfaction ratings.

The College of Veterinary Medicine blends cornfields with biotechnology and cow barns with state-of-the-art diagnostic laboratories. The college provides contemporary facilities such as Lewis Hospital for Companion Animals, built in 1983, which is one of the most modern, well-equipped veterinary teaching hospitals in the country, and the Raptor Center, which in 1988 became the world's first facility designed specifically for birds of prey. The educational opportunities extend beyond the campus to include farms throughout Minnesota and around the world. Students are given opportunities to learn about the practice of contemporary veterinary medicine through preceptorships, clinical rotations, and first-hand experiences with practitioners.

## Application Information

For specific application information (availability, deadlines, fees, and VMCAS participation), please refer to the contact information listed above.

*Residency implications:* first priority is given to Minnesota residents, minority applicants, and residents of states/provinces with which a reciprocity agreement exists (North Dakota, South Dakota, Manitoba). Residents of other states are encouraged to apply. International applicants are only considered if their preveterinary courses have been completed at a U.S. college or university.

## Prerequisites for Admission

*Course requirements and quarter hours*

| | |
|---|---|
| Freshman English, communication | 6–9 |
| Mathematics | 3–5 |
| Chemistry (with laboratory) | |
|     General inorganic | 8–12 |
|     General organic* | 5–10 |
| Biology (with laboratory) | 3–5 |
| Zoology/animal biology (with laboratory) | 3–5 |
| Physics (with laboratory) | 8–12 |
| Biochemistry | 3–5 |
| Genetics | 3–5 |
| Microbiology (with laboratory) | 3–5 |
| Liberal education | 12–18 |

\* Two quarters with one laboratory or one semester with laboratory

A minimum of 4 courses from the following areas of study: anthropology, art, economics, geography, history, humanities, literature (including foreign language literature), music, political science, psychology, public speaking or small group (interpersonal) communication, social science, sociology, theater. No more than 2 courses can be from the same area of study.

*Required undergraduate GPA:* no minimum required. The class of 2004 had a mean GPA of 3.56 (on a 4.00 scale) for required courses and 3.64 for the last 60 quarter-hour or 45 semester-hour credits of coursework prior to admission.

*AP credit policy:* must appear on official college transcripts and be equivalent to the appropriate college-level coursework.

*Course completion deadline:* prerequisite courses must be completed by the end of the spring term (not later than June 15) of the academic year in which application is made.

*Standardized examinations:* Graduate Record Examination (GRE), general test, is required, and results must be received by January 31. The mean combined score for the 3 tests for the class entering in fall 2000 was 1880.

## Summary of Admission Procedure

*Timetable*

Application deadline: October 1
Date acceptances mailed: late March
School begins: early September

*Deposit* (to hold place in class): $100.00 for Minnesota, Manitoba, South Dakota, and North Dakota residents; $250.00 for nonresidents.

*Deferments:* can be requested for special circumstances that warrant a 1-year delay in admission.

*Evaluation criteria*

| | |
|---|---|
| *Objective measures of educational background* | 70 points |
| GPA in required courses | 20 points |
| GPA in recent courses | 20 points |
| Test scores | 30 points |
| *Subjective measures of personal experience* | 30 points |
| Animal/veterinary knowledge, experience, and interest | |
| Employment record | |
| Communication skills | |
| Extracurricular and/or community service activities | |
| Leadership abilities | |
| References | |
| Maturity/reliability | |

*2000–2001 admissions summary*

| | Number of Applicants | Number of New Entrants |
|---|---|---|
| Resident | 152 | 61 |
| Reciprocity* | 24 | 2 |
| Nonresident | 751 | 17 |
| Total: | 927 | 80 |

The figures for new entrants include students taking delayed admission from the previous year.

*For further information, see the listing of contracting states and provinces.

## Expenses for the 2000–2001 Academic Year

*Tuition and fees*

| | |
|---|---|
| Residents and reciprocity (approximate) | $10,302.00 |
| Nonresidents | $20,572.00 |

# Mississippi State University

Office of Student Affairs
College of Veterinary Medicine
P.O. Box 9825
Mississippi State University
Mississippi State MS 39762
Telephone: (662) 325-1129
E-mail: coats@cvm.msstate.edu
www.cvm.msstate.edu

Mississippi State University is located in Starkville (population 20,000). The university has an enrollment of over 15,000. Places of historical interest are prevalent throughout the area. Temperatures are moderate, ranging from the 40s in January to the 90s in July. Air service to the area is 15 minutes away with daily flights that connect with Memphis, Atlanta, and Nashville.

Each class in the College of Veterinary Medicine has 50 students and begins with the summer semester. The curriculum involves 2 primary learning environments: a problem-based learning mode in which students learn basic and clinical sciences through exposure to simulated cases in small group settings, and an experiential mode in which students are rotated through each functional area of the veterinary teaching hospital assisting in primary diagnosis and care. Significant elective opportunities allow students the flexibility to focus study by species, species group, or discipline. A college-wide computer network coupled with a student computer requirement facilitates student communication and access to up-to-date veterinary medical information. Visitors are welcome at the College of Veterinary Medicine and are invited to telephone the Office of Student Affairs. The college suggests calling 2 weeks ahead of the proposed visit so that an appointment may be scheduled.

## Application Information

For specific application information (availability, deadlines, fees, and VMCAS participation), please refer to the contact information listed above.

*Residency implications:* Mississippi accepts up to 19 nonresident students.

## Prerequisites for Admission

Science and math courses must be on the level of those required for preveterinary, predentistry, or science majors and must be completed or updated within 6 calendar years prior to anticipated date of enrollment.

*Course requirements and semester hours*
Communication
| | |
|---|---|
| English composition | 6 |
| Oral communication | 3 |

Biological sciences, with laboratories: microbiology, 14
vertebrate zoology, cell biology, genetics

Physical sciences, with laboratories: inorganic chemistry, 18
organic chemistry, biochemistry, physics

Mathematics
College algebra, analytic geometry, trigonometry, 6
calculus, finite mathematics, or statistics

Nutrition (human or animal) 3-5

Humanities, fine arts, and social/behavioral sciences 15

*Required undergraduate GPA:* a minimum GPA of 2.80 on a 4.00 scale. The required prerequisite and science GPA is 3.00. The class of 2004 has an average undergraduate GPA of 3.59.

*AP credit policy:* must appear on official college transcripts and be equivalent to the appropriate college-level coursework.

*Course completion deadline:* prerequisites must be completed prior to matriculation in late May/early June.

*Standardized examinations:* Veterinary College Admission Test (VCAT) or Graduate Record Exam (GRE), general test.

*Additional requirements and considerations*
Evaluation of written application
Confidential evaluations
Interview (by invitation on a competitive basis)

## Summary of Admission Procedure

*Timetable*
Application deadline: October 1
Date interviews are held: late February-early March
Date acceptances mailed: mid-March
School begins: late May-early June

*Deposit* (to hold place in class): $500.00.

*Deferments:* requests are considered on an individual basis.

| Evaluation criteria | % weight |
|---|---|
| Grades | 50 |
| Test scores | 10 |
| Interview; animal/veterinary experience | 25 |
| References (3 required, one by a veterinarian) | 5 |
| Application (includes essay) | 10 |

*2000–2001 admissions summary*

| | | Number of Applicants | Number of New Entrants |
|---|---|---|---|
| Resident | | 80 | 35 |
| Nonresident | | 400 | 15 |
| | Total: | 480 | 50 |

## Expenses for the 2000–2001 Academic Year

*Tuition and fees*

| Tuition | $6,000.00 |
|---|---|
| Professional Education Fee* | $14,740.00 |
| Activities fee | $1,222.00 |

\* Assessment of the Professional Education Fee is based upon participation in the Mississippi tax system, and state of legal residency is not a factor.

## Dual-Degree Programs

Combined DVM–graduate degree programs are available.

Clinical experience is a vital and often enjoyable part of veterinary medical education. Photo courtesy of Mississippi State University College of Veterinary Medicine.

# University of Missouri

Office of Academic Affairs
College of Veterinary Medicine
W203 Veterinary Medicine Building
University of Missouri-Columbia
Columbia MO 65211
Telephone: (573) 884-6435
E-mail: seayk@missouri.edu
www.missouri.edu

The University of Missouri, with its 23,000 students, is located in Columbia, Missouri. The city of 76,000 is situated 125 miles from St. Louis and Kansas City and about 100 miles north of the Missouri Ozarks. Columbia is a city of 3 colleges, some light industry, major insurance companies, and a number of health-related facilities, including a medical school, and a veterans' hospital, in addition to the veterinary medical college.

The city and campus provide many cultural activities and sporting events. Living conditions are good, and housing is plentiful. Many students elect to live in the country, which is only a short distance from the College of Veterinary Medicine. Hunting for turkey, deer, quail, and other game is available. Fishing throughout the state ranges from farm ponds to large lakes and clear running streams. The climate is generally mild, although some parts of the summer are hot and humid. Winter may have a few days of snow or ice.

## Application Information

For specific application information (availability, deadlines, fees, and VMCAS participation), please refer to the contact information listed above.

*Residency implications:* first priority is given to Missouri residents; second priority is given to nonresidents. U.S. citizenship or permanent residency is required.

## Prerequisites for Admission

*Course requirements and semester hours*

| | |
|---|---|
| English or communication | 6 |
| College algebra or more advanced mathematics | 3 |
| Inorganic chemistry | 8 |
| Organic chemistry (with laboratory) | 5 |
| Physics | 5 |

| Biological science | 10 |
| Social sciences or humanities | 10 |
| Electives | 10 |
| Biochemistry | 3 |

*Required undergraduate GPA:* a cumulative GPA of 2.50 or more on a 4.00 scale is required for Missouri residents. Nonresidents must have a cumulative GPA of 3.00 or more. The most recent entering class had a mean GPA of 3.57 at the time of acceptance.

*AP credit policy:* not accepted unless documented on University of Missouri transcript.

*Course completion deadline:* prerequisite courses must be completed by the end of the winter semester or spring quarter of the year of entry.

*Standardized examinations:* Veterinary College Admission Test (VCAT) is required. Scores must be received by the Admissions Office by February 1. A minimum composite percentile score of 20 is required. The most recent entering class had a mean score of 66.44.

*Additional requirements and considerations*
  Animal/veterinary experience
  Recommendations/evaluations (3 required)
    Employer
    Academic advisors/faculty member
    Veterinarians
  Extracurricular and/or community service activities
  Essays
    Animal experience
    Explanation of choice of veterinary medicine as a profession
  Employment history

## Summary of Admission Procedure

*Timetable*
  Application deadline: November 1
  Date interviews are held: February–March
  Date acceptances mailed: mid-April
  School begins: late August

*Deposit* (to hold place in class): $100.00 for residents; $250.00 for nonresidents.

*Deferments:* each is considered individually by the admissions committee.

*Evaluation criteria*

The admission process consists of a file review of all applicants and a personal interview of residents only.

|  | % weight |
|---|---|
| Grades | 50 |
| Test scores | 5 |
| Animal/veterinary experience | 15 |
| Interview | 10 |
| References | 10 |
| Essay | 10 |

*2000–2001 admissions summary*

|  | Number of Applicants | Number of New Entrants |
|---|---|---|
| Resident | 158 | 54 |
| Nonresident | 59 | 10 |
| Total: | 217 | 64 |

## Expenses for the 2000–2001 Academic Year

*Tuition and fees*

| Resident | $10,570.00 |
|---|---|
| Nonresident | $20,550.00 |

## Dual-Degree Programs

Combined DVM–graduate degree programs are available.

## Early Admission Program

The Pre-veterinary Medicine Scholars Program guarantees acceptance into the professional program upon satisfactory completion of the undergraduate requirements. Eligibility requires a high-school senior or University of Missouri freshman to have a composite ACT score of at least 30, or an equivalent SAT score. Eligible applicants will be interviewed, and a satisfactory score must be achieved to become a Pre-Vet Med Scholar. Selected veterinary medical faculty will be assigned as mentors. Scholars receive priority consideration for part-time employment in the college. Further information may be obtained by contacting the Office of Academic Affairs at the address indicated on page 71.

# North Carolina State University

Student Services Office
College of Veterinary Medicine
4700 Hillsborough Street
North Carolina State University
Raleigh NC 27606
Telephone: (919) 829-6262
E:mail: karen_potter@ncsu.edu
www.cvm.ncsu.edu

The North Carolina State College of Veterinary Medicine is located on a 182-acre site in Raleigh, which has a population of more than 273,000. The sandy shores of North Carolina's beautiful coastline are a short ride to the east, and the Great Smoky Mountains are to the west. The climate includes mild winters and warm summers.

The College of Veterinary Medicine opened in the fall of 1981 and occupies more than 260,000 square feet, including a teaching hospital, classrooms, animal wards, research and teaching laboratories, and an audiovisual area. The college has 120 faculty members and a capacity for 288 veterinary medical students with training for interns, residents, and graduate students.

## Application Information

For specific application information (availability, deadlines, fees, and VMCAS participation), please refer to the contact information listed above.

*Residency implications:* priority is given to North Carolina residents. There are approximately 14 nonresident positions.

## Prerequisites for Admission

*Course requirements and semester hours*

| | |
|---|---|
| English composition I, plus either English composition II, public speaking, or communication | 6 |
| College calculus | 4 |
| Introduction to statistics | 3 |
| General physics I, II (with laboratory) | 8 |
| General chemistry I, II (with laboratory) | 8 |
| Organic chemistry I, II (with laboratory) | 8 |
| General biology (with laboratory) | 4 |
| Principles of genetics | 4 |

| General microbiology (with laboratory) | 4 |
| Biochemistry | 3 |
| Animal nutrition/animal science/animal husbandry | 3 |
| Social sciences and humanities | 6 |
| Business/finance | 6 |

*AP credit policy:* must appear on official college transcripts and be equivalent to the appropriate college-level coursework.

*Course completion deadline:* only 2 courses may be pending completion in the spring semester, and both must be completed (with transcript evidence) by the end of the spring semester prior to matriculation. Pending courses (including correspondence courses) may not be completed in summer sessions.

*Standardized examinations:* Graduate Record Examination (GRE), general test, is required. The scores must be received by the October 1 application deadline.

*Additional requirements and considerations*
    Animal/veterinary knowledge, experience, motivation, and maturity
    Personal statement
    Recommendations/evaluations (3 required; at least 2 from veterinarians)
    Extracurricular activities

## Summary of Admission Procedure

*Timetable*
    Application deadline: October 1
    Date acceptances mailed: third week in March
    School begins: August

*Deposit* (to hold place in class): $250.00.

*Deferments:* are considered for 1 year only, subject to Admissions Committee approval.

*Evaluation criteria*
Selection for admission is a 2-phase process:
    *Objective score:*
        Required course GPA
        Cumulative GPA
        GPA in last 45+ credits attempted
        Test score
    *Subjective score:*
        Folder review

*2000-2001 admissions summary*

|  |  | Number of Applicants | Number of New Entrants* |
|---|---|---|---|
| Resident |  | 217 | 62 |
| Nonresident |  | 873 | 14 |
|  | Total: | 1,090 | 76 |

\* Estimated

## Expenses for the 2000-2001 Academic Year

*Tuition and fees* (estimated)

| Resident | $4,935.00 |
|---|---|
| Nonresident | $23,000.00 |

## Dual Degree Programs

Combined DVM-graduate degree programs are available.

## Early Admission Program

Two special admissions options are available: (1) for North Carolina residents focusing on swine or poultry medicine in concert with the College of Agriculture and Life Sciences, and (2) for students focusing on laboratory animal medicine in concert with the College of Agriculture at North Carolina A&T State University.

# The Ohio State University

Chairperson, Admissions Committee
College of Veterinary Medicine
0004 Veterinary Hospital
601 Tharp Street
The Ohio State University
Columbus OH 43210-1089
Telephone: (614) 292-8831
Fax: (614) 262-6989
E:mail: fenner.2@osu.edu
www.vet.ohio-state.edu/docs/

Ohio State University is located in Columbus, the capital of Ohio. Columbus is a congregation of cities and villages with a sense of history and a friendly atmosphere. The third-ranking center of scientific and technological research and data dissemination in the United States, the city offers fine arts, restaurants, sports, architecture, nature, community festivals, churches, and other areas of interest.

The Ohio State University is one of the nation's leading academic centers, with a sprawling campus straddling the Olentangy River. The campus consists of thousands of acres, hundreds of buildings, more than 15,000 faculty and staff, and more than 54,000 students. The veterinary college is the third-oldest in the United States and is one of the largest veterinary colleges in North America. The patient load is one of the highest in the country, and farmlands can be accessed 10 miles from campus. The faculty members have diverse academic and research activities, and 85 percent of the clinical teaching faculty are board certified. The academic curriculum is a 4-year program that blends some clinical experience into the first 2 years, while the last 2 years are mostly clinical.

## Application Information

For specific application information (availability, deadlines, fees, and VMCAS participation), please refer to the contact information listed above.

*Residency implications:* priority is given to Ohio residents. Ohio contracts with West Virginia (5). Ohio will consider qualified nonresident students.

## Prerequisites for Admission

For the humanities and social sciences requirement, students are encouraged to elect the courses required for the bachelor of science curriculum. Courses in communication, journalism, sociology, economics, and animal behavior are strongly recommended.

Students enrolled in the preveterinary medicine curriculum are encouraged to take electives that will provide a well-rounded education in addition to those biological sciences preparatory to the veterinary medical curriculum.

*Course requirements and quarter hours*

| | |
|---|---|
| English | 5 |
| General chemistry (with laboratory)* | 15 |
| Organic chemistry* | 6 |
| Biochemistry* | 5 |
| Biology* | 10 |
| Genetics* | 5 |
| Microbiology (with laboratory)* | 5 |
| Mathematics (algebra and trigonometry) | 5 |
| General physics (with laboratory) | 10 |
| Humanities and social sciences | 20 |
| Electives | 10 |

\* Must have been completed within the 10 years preceding the application deadline.

Graduate students must have a letter from their advisor releasing them from their graduate program if accepted into the veterinary medicine program.

*Required undergraduate GPA:* the minimum acceptable GPA for Ohio residents is 2.80; however, students with 3.00 average or above will be given preferential consideration. The minimum acceptable GPA for contract-state residents is 3.00 and for nonresidents is 3.40 (on a 4.00 scale). An undergraduate degree is not a requirement. A single, comprehensive GPA, which will include grades from all college-level work (both graduate and undergraduate) completed by the applicant, is calculated.

*AP credit policy:* not available.

*Course completion deadline:* all but one prerequisite course must be completed by the end of the fall semester or quarter coinciding with submission of the application. The final remaining prerequisite course must be completed at the end of the following term (spring semester or winter quarter). Failure to satisfactorily complete prerequisites will result in automatic loss of a candidate's seat in the class.

*Standardized examinations:* Scores from one of the following standardized examinations must be submitted at the time of application:

Graduate Record Examination (GRE): minimum acceptable score 1500 total of all three subtests.

Medical College Admission Test (MCAT): minimum acceptable score 24 total; score O-T on essay portion (new MCAT).

Veterinary College Admission Test (VCAT): minimum acceptable score 50th percentile.

Scores must not be older than five years prior to the application year. The most recent acceptable date for taking the examination is September 30 of the application year.

*Additional requirements and considerations*

Minimum of 50 hours work with a veterinarian (volunteer or paid)
Academic improvement/difficulty
Personal evaluations
Involvement in community affairs
Communication/interpersonal skills
Initiative/leadership
Attitude/motivation/judgment
Work record/financial responsibility
Social and personal support systems
Comprehensiveness of veterinary medical/animal work experience
Comparative medical experience

## Summary of Admission Procedure

*Timetable*

Application deadline: October 1
Date interviews are held: November–March
Date acceptances mailed: December–March
School begins: late September

*Deposit* (to hold place in class): $25.00 for residents; $300.00 for contract and nonresident applicants.

*Deferments:* not considered.

*Evaluation criteria*

|  | % weight |
|---|---|
| Grades | 35 |
| Test scores | 10 |
| Interview* | 55 |

\* Preferred applicants are interviewed and evaluated by members of the Admissions Committee. The academic interview covers subjective areas such as academic improvement versus difficulty, communication/interpersonal skills, involvement in social and community activities, social and personal support systems, work record/financial responsibility, motivation and commitment to veterinary medicine, comprehension of veterinary medicine, knowledge of and/or exposure to animals, and references. Those applicants given the highest overall evaluation are selected for the entering class.

*2000-2001 admissions summary*

|  | Number of Applicants | Number of New Entrants |
|---|---|---|
| Resident | 302 | 95 |
| Contract* | 42 | 6 |
| Nonresident | 595 | 34 |
| Total: | 939 | 135 |

## Expenses for the 2000-2001 Academic Year

*Tuition and fees*

| Resident | $11,076.00 |
|---|---|
| Nonresident† | $31,440.00 |

\* For further information, see the listing of contracting states and provinces.

† Contract students are assessed the nonresident tuition and fees. The contract state subsidy is subtracted from that tuition, and the student pays the balance due.

## Dual-Degree Programs

Combined DVM-graduate degree programs are available.

# Oklahoma State University

Admissions Office
College of Veterinary Medicine
Oklahoma State University
Stillwater OK 74078-2003
Telephone: (405) 744-6653
Fax: (405) 744-0356
E-mail: vmadmps@okstate.edu
www.okstate.edu

Oklahoma State University is located in Stillwater, which has a population of about 42,000. Stillwater is in north central Oklahoma about 65 miles from Oklahoma City and 69 miles from Tulsa. The campus is exceptionally beautiful, with modified Georgian-style architecture in the new buildings. It encompasses 840 acres and more than 60 major academic buildings.

Three major buildings form the veterinary medicine complex. The oldest, McElroy Hall, houses the William E. Brock Memorial Library and Learning Center, as well as new classrooms and laboratories. The Boren Veterinary Medical Teaching Hospital provides the most modern facilities for both academic and clinical instruction. Completing the triad is the Oklahoma Animal Disease Laboratory, which provides both teaching resources and services to Oklahoma agriculture and industry. The College of Veterinary Medicine is fully accredited by the American Veterinary Medical Association. Faculty members in the 3 academic departments share responsibility for the curriculum. These departments are Veterinary Clinical Sciences, Veterinary Pathobiology, and Physiological Sciences.

## Application Information

For specific application information (availability, deadlines, fees, and VMCAS participation), please refer to the contact information listed above.

*Residency implications:* priority is given to Oklahoma residents. Nonresidents may apply, and Oklahoma State could admit up to 4 contract students from New Jersey and up to 14 first-time nonresident students (including any contract students from Arkansas).

## Prerequisites for Admission

*Course requirements and semester hours*

| | |
|---|---|
| English composition | 6 |
| English elective | 2 |
| General chemistry (with laboratory) | 8 |
| Organic chemistry (with laboratory) | 8 |
| Biochemistry | 3 |
| Physics | 8 |
| Mathematics | 3 |
| Zoology (with laboratory) | 4 |
| Animal nutrition | 3 |
| Biological science elective | 3 |
| Microbiology (with laboratory) | 4 |
| Genetics (laboratory recommended) | 3 |
| Humanities or social sciences | 6 |
| Electives (science or business) | 2 |

*Required undergraduate GPA:* a minimum GPA of 2.80 on a 4.00 scale is required in prerequisite courses. The mean cumulative GPA of the 2000 entering class was 3.49.

*AP credit policy:* not available.

*Alternative admissions:* in the interest of social justice and cultural diversity, the Oklahoma State Regents for Higher Education permit the college to accept up to 15 percent of a beginning class who do not meet minimum requirements. Limited to Oklahoma residents.

*Course completion deadline:* prerequisite courses must be completed by the end of the spring semester just prior to matriculation.

*Standardized examinations:* Graduate Record Examination (GRE), general test and biology subject test, is required. Earliest acceptable test date is June 1997. The class of 2004 had mean scores of 476 verbal, 588 quantitative, 627 analytical, and 566 biology.

*Additional requirements and considerations*

Evidence of motivation over an extended period of time
Animal/veterinary work experience
Amount of undergraduate education completed
Recommendations/evaluations (3 required)
    Academic advisor, preferred
    Employer
    Veterinarian

Demonstrated leadership and interpersonal skills

All science courses must have been taken within the past 8 years of application (fall 1993)

## Summary of Admission Procedure

*Timetable*
Application deadline: October 1
Date interviews held: February
Date acceptances mailed: March
School begins: mid- to late August

*Deposit* (to hold place in class): resident, $100.00; nonresident, $500.00.

*Deferments:* to complete graduate degree, deferments are considered.

*Evaluation criteria*
The admission procedure consists of evaluation of both academic and nonacademic criteria. The Admissions Committee considers all factors in the applicant's file, but the following are especially important: academic ability; familiarity with the profession and sincerity of interest; recommendations; test scores; extracurricular activities; character, personality, and general fitness and commitment for a career in veterinary medicine. The committee selects those applicants considered most capable of excelling as veterinary medical students and who possess the greatest potential for success in veterinary medicine.

*2000-2001 admissions summary*

|  |  | Number of Applicants | Number of New Entrants |
|---|---|---|---|
| Resident |  | 112 | 56 |
| Nonresident |  | 340 | 18 |
|  | Total: | 452 | 74 |

## Expenses for the 2000-2001 Academic Year

*Tuition and fees*
Resident                    $7,300.00
Nonresident                 $19,200.00

## Dual-Degree Programs
Combined DVM-graduate degree programs are available.

# Oregon State University

Office of the Dean
College of Veterinary Medicine
Oregon State University
200 Magruder Hall
Corvallis OR 97331-4801
Telephone: (541) 737-2098
Fax: (541) 737-4245
E-mail: cvmproginfo@orst.edu
www.vet.orst.edu

At Oregon State University's College of Veterinary Medicine, students learn the skills to treat and prevent animal diseases through a rigorous course of study taught by a dedicated faculty.

The city of Corvallis, home of OSU, is a modern city of approximately 50,000 that boasts theaters and parks, an art center and shopping malls, and public transportation and bicycle paths to every corner of the community. Life in Corvallis includes lectures, concerts, films, and exhibits through the university. Students can explore the great outdoors just over an hour away by car at the spectacular Oregon coast, the snow-capped Oregon Cascades, and the city of Portland. In the heart of the agriculturally rich Willamette River Valley, Corvallis enjoys colorful and crisp autumns, mild and rainy winters, flowering springs, and warm, dry summers.

Each year, OSU accepts 28 students from Oregon and a total of 8 students from the western regional contract states (Arizona, Hawaii, Montana, Nevada, New Mexico, North Dakota, Utah, and Wyoming) and all other states except Washington and Idaho. The first year of professional study is at OSU. Students then transfer to Washington State University in Pullman for the second year and half of the third year of study; then return to Corvallis to complete the remainder of their third year and also their fourth and final year of professional instruction. The small class size and the shared approach to veterinary medical education, unique in the United States, helps to provide the students with an excellent veterinary education and the opportunity to interact with faculty and students of 2 prestigious veterinary colleges.

## Application Information

For specific application information (availability, deadlines, fees, and VMCAS participation), please refer to the contact information listed above.

*Residency implications:* Oregon residents and WICHE-sponsored students are eligible for resident fees. A limited number of students are accepted as non-residents.

## Prerequisites for Admission

*Course requirements and quarter hours*

| | |
|---|---|
| Chemistry | A sequence of inorganic chemistry with laboratories; organic chemistry sufficient to meet requirements for upper-division biochemistry course or course sequence; and at least one upper-division biochemistry course |
| Mathematics | Sufficient to meet the prerequisite for physics and inorganic chemistry (at least college-level algebra) |
| Physics | 2 quarters or 1 semester of college-level physics for science majors |
| Zoology or biology | 1 year sequence |
| Genetics | 1 quarter or semester |
| Biological sciences | A minimum of at least 6 additional quarter hours or 4 semester hours of upper-division biological science courses, with at least one laboratory (physiology, cell physiology, cell biology, microbiology, or additional biochemistry) |

Total minimum number of credits required: 107 quarter credits; 72 semester credits.

*Required undergraduate GPA:* overall GPA must be at least 3.00 or the last 2 years must be at least 3.00. The mean overall GPA for the class entering in fall of 2000 was 3.54.

*AP credit policy:* must appear on official college transcripts and be equivalent to the appropriate college-level coursework.

*Course completion deadline:* prerequisite courses must be completed by June 15 prior to entry.

*Standardized examinations:* Graduate Record Examination (GRE), general test, is required. The most recent acceptable test date for applicants to the class of 2006 is November 30, 2001. The mean score of the 2000 entering class was at the 61.91 percentile.

*Additional requirements and considerations:*

Animal/veterinary work experience: applicants must have some veterinary medical exposure and animal work experience by November 1 of the year of application to be considered for admission. Working with veterinarians is the most common approach to fulfilling this requirement. Some credit will be given for animal experience such as breeding, rearing, feeding, and showing various species of animals, including companion animals, livestock, laboratory animals, zoo animals, or wildlife. Experience in veterinary clinics and hospitals and in research laboratories is highly encouraged.

Recommendations (3 required, one by a veterinarian)

Extracurricular and/or community service activities desirable

## Summary of Admission Procedure

*Timetable*

Application deadline: November 1

Date interviews are held: late February to early March

Date acceptances mailed: mid-March

School begins: late September

*Deposit* (to hold place in class): $50.00

*Deferments:* are rare.

*Evaluation criteria*

The admission procedure consists of 2 parts: a file review and a personal interview of applicants considered to be competitive. (Interviews for non-residents and WICHE students may not be required.)

|  | *% weight* |
|---|---|
| Grades | 30 |
| Test scores | 6 |
| Animal/veterinary experience | 16 |
| Interview | 22 |
| References, personal development | 21 |
| Academic index: quality and quantity of course load, work commitments, etc. | 5 |

(Additional points may be awarded in a "diversity/adversity" category.)

*2000-2001 admissions summary*

|  | Number of Applicants | Number of New Entrants |
|---|---|---|
| Resident | 103 | 28 |
| Contract (WICHE)* | 202 | 1 |
| Nonresident | 724 | 7 |
| Total: | 1,029 | 36 |

## Expenses for the 2000-2001 Academic Year

*Tuition and fees*

| | |
|---|---|
| Resident (approximate) | $10,860.00 |
| Nonresident | |
|   Contract* | $10,860.00 |
|   Other nonresident (approximate) | $21,159.00 |

\* For further information, see the listing of contracting states and provinces.

## Dual-Degree Programs

Combined DVM-graduate degree programs are available.

# University of Pennsylvania

Admissions Office
School of Veterinary Medicine
3800 Spruce Street
University of Pennsylvania
Philadelphia PA 19104-6044
Telephone: (215) 898-5434
E-mail: admissions@vet.upenn.edu
www.vet.upenn.edu

The University of Pennsylvania is located in West Philadelphia. Philadelphia is a city with a strong cultural heritage. Independence National Park includes 1 square mile of historic Philadelphia next to the Delaware River. Included are Independence Hall, the Liberty Bell, and many fine examples of colonial architecture. Philadelphia also offers theaters, museums, sports, and outdoor recreation. The Philadelphia Zoo, first in the nation, houses more than 1,600 mammals, birds, reptiles, and amphibians. The School of Veterinary Medicine enjoys a close relationship with the zoo.

The School of Veterinary Medicine was founded in 1884 and includes a hospital for small animals, classrooms, and research facilities in the city. The large-animal hospital and research facilities are located at the New Bolton Center, an 800-acre farm 40 miles west of Philadelphia. The first 2 years are spent on the main campus. Part of the third year may be spent at the New Bolton Center, and the fourth year is spent in rotation and on electives at varying campus locations. Off-campus electives are frequently permitted.

## Application Information

For specific application information (availability, deadlines, fees, and VMCAS participation), please refer to the contact information listed above.

*Residency implications:* priority is given to Pennsylvania residents. Contract arrangements are with New Jersey. The number of nonresident places is usually 45–50, including international applicants.

## Prerequisites for Admission

At least 3 English credits must be in composition; biology courses must provide background in genetics. Organic chemistry must cover aliphatic and aromatic compounds to fulfill the requirement.

*Course requirements and semester hours*

| | |
|---|---|
| English (including 1 writing course) | 6 |
| Physics (with laboratory) | 8 |
| Chemistry (with at least 1 laboratory) | |
| General | 8 |
| Organic | 4 |
| Biology or zoology (3 courses) | 9 |
| Social sciences or humanities | 6 |
| Calculus | 3 |
| Electives | 46 |

(Although not required, biochemistry is strongly recommended.)

*Required undergraduate GPA:* no specific GPA. Applicants are evaluated comparatively and should have at least a GPA of 3.30 to be competitive. The mean cumulative GPA of the class admitted in 2000 was 3.50.

*AP credit policy:* must appear on official college transcripts and count toward degree.

*Course completion deadline:* prerequisite courses must be completed by the end of the summer term of the year in which admission is sought.

*Standardized examinations:* Graduate Record Examination (GRE), general test, is required. Scores should be received no later than December 1. The class admitted in 2000 had an average of 575 on the verbal subtest and 700 on the quantitative subtest.

*Additional requirements and considerations*

Animal/veterinary work experience: experience working with animals, direct veterinary work, or research experience is desired. No minimum time limit. Experience should be sufficient to convince the admissions committee of motivation, interest, and understanding.

Recommendations/evaluations: 3 required, one from an academic science source; and one from a veterinarian. The third is the choice of the applicant.

Extracurricular/community service activities: additional activities in this category can provide information important to the admissions committee.

Leadership: evidence of leadership abilities is desirable.

## Summary of Admission Procedure

*Timetable*
    Application deadline: October 1
    Date interviews are held: Fridays from late January until completion
    Date acceptances mailed: within 14 days after interview
    School begins: early September

*Deposit* (to hold place in class): $500.00.

*Deferments:* are considered on an individual basis.

*Evaluation criteria*
The University of Pennsylvania accepts about 30 percent of each class without interview. The remaining seats are filled through a 2-part admission procedure, which includes a file review and personal interviews.

    Grades
    Test scores
    Animal/veterinary experience
    Interview
    References
    Essay
    English skills (TOEFL)

File review: files are reviewed in January by pairs of members of the admissions committee (including an alumni member), and decisions are made on whether or not to offer an interview.

Personal interviews: interviews are held on Fridays from late January until the class is filled. The number of interviews granted equals 2 to 3 times the number of seats available.

Two personal interviews are conducted: a formal interview with 2 faculty members (including an alumni member) of the committee, and an informal interview with student committee members. Although students do not vote on acceptance, they have a significant part in the meeting following interviews.

*2000–2001 admissions summary*

|  | Number of Applicants | Number of New Entrants |
|---|---|---|
| Resident | 233 | 56 |
| Nonresident* | 1,223 | 63 |
| Total: | 1,456 | 119 |

\* For further information, see listing of contracting states and provinces.

## Expenses for the 2000-2001 Academic Year

*Tuition and fees*

| | |
|---|---|
| Resident | $24,220.00 |
| Nonresident | |
| Contract* | $24,220.00 |
| Other nonresident | $28,800.00 |

\* For further information, see listing of contracting states and provinces.

## Dual-Degree Programs

Combined DVM–graduate degree programs are available.

# Purdue University

Student Services Office
School of Veterinary Medicine
1240 Lynn Hall
Purdue University
West Lafayette IN 47907-1240
Telephone: (765) 494-7893 or (800) 213-2859 (long distance)
E-mail: admissions@vet.purdue.edu
www.vet.purdue.edu

Purdue University is located in one of the largest metropolitan centers in northwestern Indiana. Greater Lafayette occupies a site on the Wabash River 65 miles northwest of Indianapolis and 126 miles southeast of Chicago. The combined population of the twin cities, Lafayette and West Lafayette, exceeds 64,000. The community offers an art museum, historical museum, 1,600 acres of public parks, and more than 60 churches of all major denominations.

Purdue ranks among the 25 largest colleges and universities in the nation. Students represent all 50 states and many foreign countries. Diversity and opportunity are goals that the School of Veterinary Medicine maintains in the selection of each year's entering class. The School of Veterinary Medicine has assumed a leading position nationally and internationally in veterinary education. To better prepare individuals for veterinary medical careers in the twenty-first century, new and innovative strategies are being implemented into the curriculum.

## Application Information

For specific application information (availability, deadlines, fees, and VMCAS participation), please refer to the contact information listed above.

*Residency implications:* priority is given to Indiana residents. Approximately one-third of the class will be nonresident students in a total class of 60. Applicants from all states will be considered. Purdue has no contract positions. International applicants will be considered provided both the academic and financial criteria can be met.

## Prerequisites for Admission

The course requirements outlined below are considered the bare minimum prerequisite courses to be completed. No less than a grade of C must be received in each required course in order to be considered eligible for admission.

In the electives category, humanities include languages, cognitive sciences, and social sciences; business writing and macroeconomics courses are highly recommended. Other courses that are highly recommended include computer, basic and comparative nutrition, and general animal science courses.

*Course requirements and semester hours*

| | |
|---|---|
| English composition | 6 |
| Speech (public speaking) | 3 |
| Biology (with laboratory) (diversity, development, cell structure) | 8–13 |
| Chemistry, general (with laboratory) | 8–10 |
| Chemistry, organic (with laboratory) or chemistry, organic (with laboratory) (1 semester) and quantitative analysis (1 semester) | 8–9 |
| Biochemistry | 3–6 |
| Calculus | 6–10 |
| Physics (with laboratory) | 8 |
| Genetics (with laboratory) | 4 |
| Statistics | 3 |
| Humanities | 9 |

*Required undergraduate GPA:* the mean cumulative GPA of the 2000 entering class was 3.56 on a 4.00 scale. The minimum overall GPA required for consideration is 3.00 on a 4.00 scale for nonresident applicants.

*AP credit policy:* must appear on official college transcripts and be equivalent to the appropriate college-level coursework.

*Course completion deadline:* minimum prerequisite courses must be completed by the end of the spring term prior to matriculation.

*Standardized examinations:* Graduate Record Examination (GRE), general test, is required. Test scores must be received no later than December 1 of the year of application.

*Additional requirements and considerations*
  Animal/veterinary experience
  Amount of college education
  Recommendations/evaluations (3 required)
    Academic advisor/faculty member
    Employer
    Veterinarian
  Essay
  Employment record
  Extracurricular college experience

## Summary of Admission Procedure

*Timetable*
  Application deadline: October 1
  Date interviews are held: February
  Date acceptances mailed: March
  School begins: late August

*Deposit* (to hold place in class): $250.00 for residents; $1,000.00 for nonresidents.

*Deferments:* request for deferments will be considered on a case-by-case basis.

*Evaluation criteria*
The admission process consists of:
    A preliminary review based upon grade point indices, test scores, and
      prerequisite course completion
    An in-depth review of selected applicants
    A personal interview by invitation

| | *% weight* |
|---|---|
| Grades, test scores, overall academic performance | 50 |
| Animal, veterinary, and general work experiences, extracurricular activities, essay, overall presentation of application materials, references, and interview | 50 |

*2000-2001 admissions summary*

| | Number of Applicants | Number of New Entrants |
|---|---|---|
| Resident | 123 | 39 |
| Nonresident | 438 | 31 |
| International | 12 | 0 |
| Total: | 573 | 70 |

94

**Expenses for the 2000–2001 Academic Year**

*Tuition and fees*
| | |
|---|---|
| Resident | $8,908.00 |
| Nonresident | $21,480.00 |

**Dual-Degree Programs**

Combined DVM–graduate degree programs are available.

**Early Admission Program**

The Veterinary Scholars Program provides an opportunity for early admission into the professional program by accepting high-school seniors who

1. ranked in the top 10 percent of their graduating class;
2. have attained a combined SAT score equal to or greater than 1300 or composite ACT score equal to or greater than 28;
3. were admitted to Purdue University in animal sciences, biochemistry, or biological sciences programs; and
4. demonstrate a background of work experience with animals and veterinarians.

Students admitted to the program must complete all preveterinary prerequisite coursework, obtain a bachelor's degree with stipulated grade point averages for each year of undergraduate study, and submit scores from the GRE (Graduate Record Exam), general test, and the GRE Writing Assessment test during their senior year.

Students following the equine and companion-animal tracks at Purdue University's School of Veterinary Medicine enjoy the facilities of the Equine Sports Medicine Center. Photo by Vincent P. Walter, courtesy of Purdue University.

# University of Tennessee

Office of the Associate Dean
College of Veterinary Medicine
P.O. Box 1071
University of Tennessee
Knoxville TN 37901-1071
Telephone: (865) 974-7263
E-mail: jbrace@utk.edu
www.vet.utk.edu

The University of Tennessee's College of Veterinary Medicine is located in Knoxville, a city of 175,000 situated in the Appalachian foothills of east central Tennessee. Only 45 minutes from the Great Smoky Mountains National Park and 3 hours from both Nashville and Atlanta, Knoxville offers many recreational and cultural opportunities, including a symphony orchestra, an opera company, and several fine theaters. The climate in Knoxville is moderate with distinct seasons.

The 417-acre Knoxville campus of the University of Tennessee has about 20,010 undergraduate and 5,464 graduate students. The modern Clyde M. York Veterinary Medicine Building, housing the teaching and research facilities, Veterinary Teaching Hospital, and Agriculture-Veterinary Medicine Library, faces the Tennessee River on the university's Agricultural Campus.

The curriculum of the College of Veterinary Medicine is a 9-semester, 4-year program. Development of a strong basic science education is emphasized in the first year. The second and third years emphasize the study of diseases, their causes, diagnosis, treatment, and prevention. Innovative features of this curriculum include 8 weeks of student-centered small-group applied-learning exercises in semesters 1–6; 3 weeks of dedicated clinical experiences in the veterinary teaching hospital in semesters 3–5; and elective course opportunities in semesters 4–6 that allow students to focus on specific educational/career goals. In the fourth year, students participate exclusively in clinical rotations in the Veterinary Teaching Hospital and required off-campus externships. The college has unique programs in zoo and exotic animal medicine and surgery, cancer diagnosis and therapy, endoscopy, and laser surgery.

## Application Information

For specific application information (availability, deadlines, fees, and VMCAS participation), please refer to the contact information listed above.

*Residency implications:* priority is given to Tennessee residents. Tennessee has no contractual agreements and does accept nonresident applications.

## Prerequisites for Admission

*Course requirements and semester hours*

| | |
|---|---|
| General inorganic chemistry (with laboratory) | 8 |
| Organic chemistry (with laboratory) | 8 |
| General biology/zoology (with laboratory) | 8 |
| Cellular biology* | 3 |
| Genetics | 3 |
| Biochemistry (exclusive of laboratory)[†] | 4 |
| Physics (with laboratory) | 8 |
| English composition | 6 |
| Social sciences/humanities | 18 |

\* Applicants are strongly encouraged to complete additional biological science courses, especially comparative anatomy, mammalian physiology, and microbiology with laboratory.

† This should be a complete upper-division course in general cellular and comparative biochemistry. Half of a 2-semester sequence will not satisfy this requirement.

*AP credit policy:* must appear on official college transcripts and be equivalent to the appropriate college-level coursework.

*Required undergraduate GPA:* for nonresident applicants, the minimum acceptable cumulative GPA is 3.20 on a 4.00 scale. At time of acceptance, the mean GPA of the class entering in fall of 2000 was 3.56.

*Course completion deadline:* prerequisite courses must be completed with a grade of C or better by the end of the spring term prior to entry.

*Standardized examinations:* Veterinary College Admission Test (VCAT) is required. For applicants planning to matriculate in August 2002, the oldest acceptable VCAT scores are from the October 1999 test date.

*Additional requirements and considerations*

Animal/veterinary work experience
Recommendations/evaluations
Extracurricular and/or community service activities
Leadership skills
Autobiographical essay (personal statement)

## Summary of Admission Procedure

*Timetable*
  Application deadline: November 1
  Date interviews are held: mid- to late March
  Date acceptances mailed: no later than April 1
  Applicant's response date: April 15
  School begins: late August

*Deposit* (to hold place in class): none required.

*Deferments:* are considered on a case-by-case basis.

*Evaluation criteria*
The admission procedure consists of an initial file review followed by an interview of selected applicants.

  Grades $\Big\}$ Initial academic file review.
  Test scores
  Animal/veterinary experience
  Interview
  References (3 required)
  Essay

*2000–2001 admissions summary*

|  | | Number of Applicants | Number of New Entrants |
|---|---|---|---|
| Resident | | 130 | 61 |
| Nonresident | | 214 | 7 |
| | Total: | 344 | 68 |

## Expenses for the 2000–2001 Academic Year

*Tuition and fees*
  Resident                         $7,060.00
  Nonresident                  $18,804.00

# Texas A & M University

Office of the Dean
College of Veterinary Medicine
Texas A & M University
College Station TX 77843-4461
Telephone: (979) 845-5038
www.cvm.tamu.edu

The university is located adjacent to the cities of Bryan and College Station. The 2 cities have a combined population of about 100,000. The student population at Texas A & M is more than 40,000. The College of Veterinary Medicine is one of the 10 original veterinary teaching institutions that existed in the United States prior to World War II.

## Application Information

For specific application information (availability, deadlines, fees, and VMCAS participation), please refer to the contact information listed above.

*Residency implications:* Texas has no contractual agreements with other states. Applicants from other states who have outstanding credentials will be considered. Successful candidates who are awarded competitive university-based scholarships may attend at resident tuition rate.

## Prerequisites for Admission

The minimum number of college or university credits required for admission into the professional curriculum is 64 semester hours. Applicants must have completed or have in progress approximately 48 credit hours at the time of application. Because there is no specific degree plan associated with preveterinary education, students are encouraged to pursue a degree plan that meets individual interests. Students are strongly encouraged to choose courses with the assistance of a knowledgeable counselor at the undergraduate institution or through contact with an academic advisor at the College of Veterinary Medicine, telephone: (979) 845-5038 or (979) 862-1169.

*Course requirements and semester hours*

*Life sciences*

| | |
|---|---|
| General biology (with laboratory) | 4 |
|     Survey of contemporary biology that covers the chemical basis of life, structure and biology of the cell, molecular biology, and genetics | |
| General microbiology (with laboratory) | 4 |
|     Basic microbiology; comparative morphology, taxonomy, pathogenesis, ecology, variation, and physiology of microorganisms | |
| Genetics | 3 |
|     Basic concepts of mammalian genetics | |
| Animal nutrition or feeds and feeding | 3 |
|     Emphasis on basic principles of animal nutrition; nutritional roles of carbohydrates, proteins, lipids, minerals, vitamins, and water; emphasis on digestion, absorption, metabolism, and excretion of the nutrients and their metabolites | |

*Chemical-physical sciences and mathematics*

| | |
|---|---|
| Inorganic chemistry (with laboratory) | 8 |
|     Basic concepts of modern inorganic chemistry | |
| Organic chemistry (with laboratory) | 4 |
|     Basic concepts of modern organic chemistry | |
| Biochemistry | 3 |
|     An introduction to the chemistry and metabolism of biologically important molecules, the biochemical basis of life processes, and cellular metabolism and regulation | |
| Calculus/statistics | 3 |
| Physics (with laboratory) | 8 |
|     Fundamentals of mechanics, heat, sound, electricity, and light | |

*Nonscience*

| | |
|---|---|
| Composition and rhetoric | 3 |
| Literature | 3 |
| Speech communication | 3 |
| Technical writing | 3 |

*Additional credits*

In addition to the 52 credit hours recommended above, an applicant must complete a minimum of 12 additional credits. Applicants should keep in mind their degree program, the core curriculum requirements for a baccalaureate degree at Texas A & M University, and their personal career goals in making these choices. Applicants are strongly encouraged to make these choices with a qualified counselor at their institution.

*Required undergraduate GPA:* the minimum overall GPA required is 2.90 on a 4.00 scale or 3.10 for the last 45 semester credits. The mean of the most recent entering class was 3.60.

*AP credit policy:* not available.

*Course completion deadline:* required courses must be completed by the end of the spring term prior to entry.

*Standardized examinations:* Graduate Record Examination (GRE), general test, is required. Standardized test scores must be 5 years old or less. The class entering in 2000 averaged 1861 (combined verbal, quantitative, and analytical subtests) on the GRE.

*Additional requirements and considerations*
Evaluations
Animal/veterinary work experience

Knowledge and experience in working with animals is crucial to becoming a successful veterinarian. While the professional curriculum is almost totally devoted to the understanding of animals, animal contact, experience, and handling should also be major considerations in the preveterinary training period. Applicants are expected to be familiar with animal systems and behavior. For those interested in farm animal veterinary medicine, general agriculture knowledge should also be a major consideration. To obtain this experience, applicants should either register for coursework based on their background, interests, and needs, or involve themselves in practical animal operations in the private sector. If designated courses in the animal sciences are not available at the applicant's institution, demonstrable experience with animals is acceptable. Formal training in animal systems and animal behavior is highly desirable and encouraged if available at the applicant's institution.

## Summary of Admission Procedure

*Timetable*
Application deadline: October 1
Date interviews are held: before February 15
Date acceptances mailed: March
School begins: late August

*Deposit* (to hold place in class): none required.

*Deferments:* requests for deferments will be considered on a case-by-case basis.

*Evaluation criteria*
Academic performance
Test scores
Interview
Personal statement
Personal evaluations (3 evaluations are required)
Semester course load and postacademic challenge
Leadership and experience

*2000–2001 admissions summary*

|  | Number of Applicants | Number of New Entrants |
|---|---|---|
| Resident | 389 | 126 |
| Nonresident | 480 | 2 |
| Total: | 869 | 128 |

## Expenses for the 2000–2001 Academic Year

*Tuition and fees*
Resident                    $8,568.00
Nonresident              $19,368.00

# Tufts University

Office of Admissions
School of Veterinary Medicine
200 Westboro Road
Tufts University
North Grafton MA 01536
Telephone: (508) 839-7920
E-mail: vetadmissions@tufts.edu
www.tufts.edu/vet/

Tufts University is located near Boston, where athletic and cultural activities abound. The School of Veterinary Medicine provides an exciting biomedical environment for the study of modern veterinary medicine. Signature programs include wildlife medicine, equine sports medicine, international veterinary medicine, biotechnology and veterinary medicine, and the study of issues related to ethical dimensions of veterinary medicine, including animal welfare.

Hands-on learning begins in the first year with a course on clinical skills and animal behavior and continues throughout the next 3 years. Many opportunities exist outside of formal courses for hands-on work in hospitals and research laboratories. The Hospital for Large Animals, Foster Hospital for Small Animals, the Ambulatory Clinic, and the Wildlife Clinic provide a rich mixture of horses, cats, dogs, cattle, sheep, goats, and native wildlife.

## Application Information

For specific application information (availability, deadlines, fees, and VMCAS participation), please refer to the contact information listed above.

*Residency implications:* Massachusetts residents make up about half of each class. All others considered for the remaining spaces. Tufts contracts with Maine (1), New Hampshire (1-2), and New Jersey (6).

## Prerequisites for Admission

*Course requirements and semesters*

| | |
|---|---|
| Biology (with laboratory) | 2 |
| Inorganic chemistry (with laboratory) | 2 |
| Organic chemistry (with laboratory) | 2 |
| Physics | 2 |
| Mathematics | 2 |
| Genetics, unless included in biology | 1 |
| Biochemistry | 1 |
| English composition | 2 |
| Social and behavioral sciences | 2 |
| Humanities and fine arts | 2 |

*Required undergraduate GPA:* no minimum GPA required. The average GPA for the class admitted in 2000 was 3.45.

*AP credit policy:* must appear on official college transcripts and be equivalent to the appropriate college-level coursework.

*Course completion deadline:* prerequisite courses must be completed by the time of matriculation into the DVM program.

*Standardized examinations:* Graduate Record Examination (GRE), general test, is required. The most recent acceptable test date for applicants to the class of 2006 is November 2001. The oldest acceptable scores must be within 5 years of the application deadline. Average GRE scores for the class of 2004 were verbal 600, quantitative 690, and analytical 720.

*Additional requirements and considerations*
- Animal/veterinary/biomedical research experience
- Recommendations/evaluations (3 required)
  - advisor/faculty members
  - veterinarian/research scientist/project leader
- Essays
- Interview

## Summary of Admission Procedure

*Timetable*
- Application deadline: December 1
- Date interviews are held: February
- Date acceptances mailed: March
- School begins: late August

*Deposit* (to hold place in class): $500.00.

*Deferments:* requests for deferment are handled on a case-by-case basis.

*Evaluation criteria*
Tufts' admission procedure consists of a review of the application and an interview of selected applicants.

*2000–2001 admissions summary*

|  | *Number of Applicants* | *Number of New Entrants* |
|---|---|---|
| Total: | 723 | 80 |

## Expenses for the 2000–2001 Academic Year

*Tuition and fees*
| | |
|---|---|
| Resident | $24,136.00 |
| Contract* | $16,065.00 |
| Nonresident | $28,065.00 |

* For further information, see the listing of contracting states and provinces.

## Dual-Degree Program

Combined DVM–graduate degree programs are available.

# Tuskegee University

School of Veterinary Medicine, Nursing, and Allied Health
Tuskegee University
Tuskegee AL 36088
Telephone: (334) 727-8460

Tuskegee University School of Veterinary Medicine is located in Tuskegee, Alabama, a city of about 25,000. Tuskegee is located about 40 miles east of Montgomery and 40 miles west of Columbus, Georgia. Summers are hot and humid, and winters are moderate. Numerous lakes, parks, recreational facilities, and other educational institutions are located nearby.

The university was founded by Booker T. Washington in 1881, and the veterinary school was established in 1945. Seventy percent of black veterinarians in the United States received their professional training at Tuskegee. A large portion of the campus has been declared a historical site by the National Park Service.

## Application Information

For specific application information (availability, deadlines, fees, and VMCAS participation), please refer to the contact information listed above.

*Residency implications:* applications are accepted nationwide, with a minimum number of contract spaces for Kentucky (2), New Jersey (2), South Carolina (4), and West Virginia (2).

## Prerequisites for Admission

*Course requirements and semester hours*

| | |
|---|---|
| English composition/communications | 6 |
| Mathematics (algebra and trigonometry) | 6 |
| Chemistry (minimum) | |
|     Organic chemistry (with laboratory) | 4 |
|     Biochemistry (with laboratory) | 4 |
| Physics* (with laboratory) | 8 |
| Biological science | |
|     Advanced biology** | 9 |
| Free electives | 8 |
|     (advanced biological science — optional) | |
| Animal science | 9 |
|     (includes poultry and animal nutrition) | |
| Social science and humanities | 6 |
| Electives — liberal arts | 6 |

\*  One academic year

\*\* Advanced biology courses, e.g., zoology, microbiology, genetics, anatomy, physiology, and histology

*Required undergraduate GPA:* the requirement is 2.70 on a 4.00 scale.

*AP credit policy:* not available.

*Course completion deadline:* prerequisite courses must be completed by the end of the spring semester of the year of application.

*Standardized examinations:* Veterinary College Admission Test (VCAT), Medical College Admission Test (MCAT), or Graduate Record Examination (GRE), any of which must be taken within 3 years of application, is required.

## Summary of Admission Procedure

*Timetable*

    Application deadline: First Monday in December
    Date interviews are held: February–March
    Date acceptances mailed: April 15
    School begins: late August

*Deposit* (to hold place in class): $275.00.

*Deferments:* one-year deferments are offered upon written request.

*Evaluation criteria*

The following items are taken into consideration: academic record, academic trends, letters of recommendation, work experience, and test scores.

|  | *% weight* |
|---|---|
| Grades | 50 |
| Test scores | 5 |
| Animal/veterinary experience | 2 |
| Interview | 20 |
| References | 2 |
| Essay | 1 |

*2000–2001 admissions summary*

|  | *Number of Applicants* | *Number of New Entrants* |
|---|---|---|
| Resident | 35 | 7 |
| Contract* | 99 | 23 |
| Nonresident | 129 | 31 |
| Total: | 263 | 61 |

## Expenses for the 2000-2001 Academic Year

*Tuition and fees*          $12,000.00

\* For further information, see the listing of contracting states and provinces.

## Dual-Degree Programs

Combined DVM–graduate degree programs are available.

# Virginia Polytechnic Institute and State University

Admissions Coordinator
Virginia-Maryland Regional College of Veterinary Medicine
Virginia Polytechnic Institute and State University
Blacksburg VA 24061
Telephone: (540) 231-4699
Fax: (540) 231-9290
E-mail: dvmadmit@vt.edu
www.vetmed.vt.edu

The Virginia-Maryland Regional College of Veterinary Medicine is situated on 3 distinct campuses. The main campus is at Virginia Tech in Blacksburg, Virginia, a community with a population of about 40,000 situated on a high plateau in southwestern Virginia between the Blue Ridge and Allegheny Mountains. Its residents enjoy a wide range of educational, social, recreational, and cultural opportunities. In addition to the Blacksburg campus, the Equine Medical Center campus is in Leesburg, Virginia, and the University of Maryland is at College Park. The college received full accreditation in 1993 from the American Veterinary Medical Association.

In recognition of a need for veterinarians trained in both basic and clinical sciences, the college offers students the opportunity to participate in graduate studies and receive appropriate advanced training to conduct research in basic or clinical disciplines. Nearly 25 percent of the nation's veterinarians work in areas other than private practice, such as government and corporate veterinary medicine. Through the assistance of a grant from the Pew Charitable Trusts, the college has established the Center for Government and Corporate Veterinary Medicine, which is a national resource for training veterinarians for the wide variety of careers in this area of the profession.

## Application Information

For specific application information (availability, deadlines, fees, and VMCAS participation), please refer to the contact information listed above.

*Residency implications:* 50 positions are reserved for Virginia residents, and 30 positions for Maryland residents. Virginia contracts with Delaware and offers up to 3 positions for Delaware residents; the remaining positions (7–10) may be filled by nonresidents.

## Prerequisites for Admission

*Course requirements and semester hours*

| | |
|---|---|
| Biological sciences (with laboratories) | 8 |
| Organic chemistry (with laboratories) | 8 |
| Physics (with laboratories) | 8 |
| Biochemistry | 3 |
| English (composition, 3 credit hours) | 6 |
| Humanities/social science | 6 |
| Mathematics (algebra, geometry, trigonometry, calculus) | 6 |

Students must earn a C- or better in all required courses.

Science courses taken 7 or more years ago may be repeated or substituted with higher-level courses with the written consent of the admissions committee.

*Required undergraduate GPA:* to be considered for admission, applicants must have a cumulative GPA of at least 2.80 on a 4.00 scale upon completion of a minimum of 2 academic years of full-time study (60 semester/90 quarter hours) at an accredited college or university. Alternatively, a 3.30 GPA in the last 2 years (60 semester hours) will qualify a student who does not have a 2.80 GPA overall. All courses taken during this 2-year period must be junior or senior level. The mean GPA of those accepted into the class of 2003 was 3.50.

*AP credit policy:* not available.

*Course completion deadline:* required courses must be completed by the end of the spring term of the year in which matriculation occurs.

*Standardized examinations:* Graduate Record Examination (GRE) is required. For the class of 2003, the mean score on the aptitude portion (verbal, quantitative, analytical) was 1850. The oldest acceptable scores must be within 5 years of the application deadline.

*Additional requirements and considerations*

Maturity and a broad cultural perspective

Motivation and dedication to a career in veterinary medicine

Evidence of potential, and appreciation of the career opportunities for veterinarians, as indicated by:

1. Clinical veterinary experience (private practice)
2. Animal experience in addition to time spent working with a veterinarian
3. Veterinary experience outside of private clinical practice, such as research, industrial, government, and corporate settings
4. Extramural activities, achievements, honors

5. Communication skills
6. References

## Summary of Admission Procedure

*Timetable*
  Application deadline: October 1
  Date interviews are held: late February/early March
  Date acceptances mailed: early March
  School begins: mid-August

*Deposit* (to hold place in class): $450.00 for  Maryland and Virginia residents; $1,000.00 for nonresidents.

*Deferments:* case-by-case basis if a candidate has extenuating circumstances beyond his or her control.

*Evaluation criteria*
The admission procedure is comprised of an initial screening of applicants, an interview of selected applicants, and a final review of the dossiers of all interviewees.

|  | *% weight* |
|---|---|
| Academics | 50 |
|     Cumulative GPA, required science GPA, last 45 semester-hour GPA, GRE aptitude | |
| Background | 25 |
|     Related animal experience; veterinary experience; research, industrial, and commercial experience; activities, achievements, and awards; narrative and personal references | |
| Interviews | 25 |

*2000–2001 admissions summary*

|  | Number of Applicants | Number of New Entrants |
|---|---|---|
| Resident | | |
|   Maryland | 138 | 30 |
|   Virginia | 145 | 50 |
| Contract* | 15 | 3 |
| Nonresident | 696 | 7 |
| Total: | 994 | 90 |

## Expenses for the 2000–2001 Academic Year

*Tuition and fees*
| | |
|---|---|
| Resident | $8,912.00 |
| Nonresident | $22,136.00 |

## Dual-Degree Programs

Combined DVM–graduate degree programs are available.

# Washington State University

Office of Student Services
College of Veterinary Medicine
Washington State University
Pullman WA 99164-7012
Telephone: (509) 335-1532

Washington State University, which has an enrollment of 20,000, is located in southeastern Washington in the town of Pullman. This small community is surrounded by farmland yet is close to the mountains of Idaho. The area offers excellent summer and winter recreation.

The College of Veterinary Medicine at WSU was founded in 1899 and is one of the 5 oldest colleges of veterinary medicine in the country. Washington, Oregon, and Idaho (WOI) have developed a regional program in veterinary medical education that also serves Alaska, Arizona, Hawaii, Montana, Nevada, New Mexico, North Dakota, Utah, and Wyoming through the Western Interstate Commission for Higher Education (WICHE) Compact.

The DVM degree is awarded by Washington State University and Oregon State University. The University of Idaho is a full partner in the program, but Idaho students receive their DVM degrees from Washington.

## Application Information

For specific application information (availability, deadlines, fees, and VMCAS participation), please refer to the contact information listed above.

*Residency implications:* priority is given to Washington and Idaho residents. WOI contracts with WICHE states (Alaska, Arizona, Hawaii, Montana, Nevada, New Mexico, North Dakota, Utah, Wyoming) for 16 places. Washington accepts a few (approximately 5) nonresidents each year from states other than contracts listed above.

## Prerequisites for Admission

*Course requirements*

| | |
|---|---|
| Chemistry | A sequence of inorganic and organic courses with laboratories and one upper-division biochemistry course |
| Mathematics | Sufficient to meet the prerequisites for inorganic chemistry and physics plus one semester of statistics |
| Physics | 1 semester or equivalent of college-level physics for science majors |
| Zoology or biology | 1-year sequence |
| Genetics | 1 semester or equivalent |

Total minimum number of credits required is 60 semester hours or 90 quarter hours.

*Required undergraduate GPA:* none; a minimum overall GPA of 3.20 on a 4.00 scale is recommended. The class of 2004 had a mean overall GPA of 3.50 at the time of acceptance.

*AP credit policy:* must appear on official college transcripts and be equivalent to the appropriate college-level coursework.

*Course completion deadline:* prerequisite courses must be completed by June 15 prior to entry.

*Standardized examinations:* Graduate Record Examination (GRE), general test, is required. Test scores older than 5 years will not be accepted. The mean combined score on the Graduate Record Examination for the class of 2004 was at the 71st percentile.

*Additional requirements and considerations*

Animal/veterinary work experience

Recommendations (3 required, one by a veterinarian)

Extracurricular and/or community service activities

## Summary of Admission Procedure

*Timetable*

Application deadline: October 1

Date interviews are held: late February–early March

Date acceptances mailed: March–April

School begins: late August

*Deposit* (to hold place in class): none required

114

*Deferments:* are considered for financial reasons and completion of graduate degrees.

*Evaluation criteria*

Applicants will be selected based upon ability to successfully complete the program and demonstration of the qualities of a good veterinarian. Academic criteria include undergraduate, science, GRE test scores, and rigor of academic program (and quality of graduate program, if applicable). Nonacademic factors include maturity, integrity, compassion, communication skills, and a desire to contribute to society. An interview will be required for residents of Washington, Idaho, and states outside the WICHE region. WICHE applicants are ranked for WICHE funding using the same criteria above minus the interview.

*2000–2001 admissions summary\**

|  | Number of Applicants | Number of New Entrants |
|---|---|---|
| Washington | 157 | 46 |
| Idaho | 41 | 11 |
| Contract[†] | 248 | 14 |
| Nonresident | 624 | 3 |
| Total: | 1,173 | 74 |

\*   Note: see also section under Oregon State University; Oregon residents apply to Oregon State University. Oregon residents should not apply to WSU through VMCAS.

## Expenses for the 2000–2001 Academic Year

*Tuition and fees*

| | |
|---|---|
| Resident | $9,260.00 |
| Nonresident | |
| Contract[†] | $9,260.00 |
| Other nonresidents | $22,960.00 |

†   For further information, see the listing of contracting states and provinces.

# University of Wisconsin

Office of Academic Affairs
School of Veterinary Medicine
2015 Linden Drive West
University of Wisconsin-Madison
Madison WI 53706-1102
Telephone: (608) 263-2525
www.vetmed.wisc.edu.oaa/oaa.html

The University of Wisconsin is located in Madison, the state capital, which has a population of about 190,000. Consistently ranked among the nation's "most livable" cities, its hilly terrain, scattered parks, and woodlands saturate the urban setting with a friendly neighborhood atmosphere. Centered on a narrow isthmus among 4 scenic lakes, the city is a recreational paradise. The university sprawls over 900 acres along Lake Mendota and its student population is nearly 45,000. It has rated among the top 10 universities academically since 1910 and is third in the country in volume of research activity.

The School of Veterinary Medicine facility has a modern veterinary teaching hospital, modern equipment, and high-quality lab space for teaching and research. The curriculum provides a broad education in veterinary medicine with learning experiences in food animal medicine and other specialty areas. The school pioneered a unique senior rotation in ambulatory service for fourth-year students where they experience the life and work of a veterinarian specializing in large-animal medicine by working in one of 20 practices near Madison. The school has an outstanding research program with faculty in the forefront. Many faculty members have joint appointments with the College of Agriculture, the Medical School, the Regional Primate Center, the McArdle Cancer Research Institute, the National Wildlife Health Laboratory, and the North Central Dairy Forage Center. These outside links provide research and job opportunities for students.

## Application Information

For specific application information (availability, deadlines, fees, and VMCAS participation), please refer to the contact information listed above.

*Residency implications:* between 60 and 70 Wisconsin residents will be accepted. Wisconsin has no contractual agreements, but may accept 10–20 nonresidents. Applicants who can claim legal residency or domicile in more than one state should contact the school. Wisconsin has a cooperative agreement with the

Pontifical Catholic University of Puerto Rico and the University of Puerto Rico-Mayaguez (UPR-Mayaguez) annually to offer admission to up to 2 students from the Pontifical Catholic University of Puerto Rico and UPR-Mayaguez. Students from Puerto Rico considering applying to the BS/DVM Binary Program should contact the College of Sciences, Pontifical Catholic University of Puerto Rico, Estacion 6, Ponce, Puerto Rico 00732 and/or the College of Agricultural Sciences, University of Puerto Rico-Mayaguez, P.O. Box 5000, Mayaguez, PR 00681-5000.

### Prerequisites for Admission

Applicants must complete a minimum of 60 semester credits of college coursework. The 60 credits include the required 40–43 credits of coursework listed below, plus a minimum of 17 credits of elective coursework left to the student's discretion. The 17 elective credits allow the student to meet personal and academic goals and objectives while preparing for admission to veterinary school.

*Course requirements and semester hours*

| | |
|---|---|
| Biochemistry (organic chemistry must be prerequisite) | 3 |
| General biology or zoology, introductory animal biology course (with laboratory) | 5 |
| General and qualitative chemistry, 2-semester lecture series (with laboratory) | 8 |
| Organic chemistry, 1-semester lecture satisfying biochemistry prerequisite | 3 |
| English composition or journalism | 6 |

Must include completion of either of the following:
1. satisfactory score on a college English placement exam, or
2. an introductory English composition course, plus completion of one of the following:
   a. an English composition or journalism course graded on the basis of writing skills, or
   b. written evidence from instructor that writing skills were included in the grading of a specific college-level course

| | |
|---|---|
| Genetics or animal breeding, must include principles of heredity and preferably molecular mechanisms | 3 |
| General physics, 2-semester lecture series | 6 |
| Statistics, introductory course | 3 |
| Social sciences/humanities, any elective courses in social science or the humanities | 6 |

*Required undergraduate GPA:* the mean cumulative GPA of the class of 2004 is approximately 3.51 for residents and 3.44 for nonresidents.

*AP credit policy:* must appear on official college transcripts and be equivalent to the appropriate college-level coursework.

*Course completion deadline:* all coursework must be completed no later than the spring 2002 term prior to admission to the fall 2002 term.

*Standardized examinations:* Graduate Record Examination (GRE), general test, is required. The GRE may be taken no later than October 1 in the year of application. The mean score of the class of 2004 for the verbal, quantitative, and analytical portions combined is approximately 1865 for residents and 1926 for nonresidents.

*Additional requirements and considerations*
> Animal contact and work experience
> Veterinary medical experience
> Other preparatory experience
> College degrees earned
> Extracurricular activities
> Recommendations/evaluations (3 required)
> Scholarships/awards

## Summary of Admission Procedure

*Timetable*
> Application deadline: October 1
> Interviews: none
> Date acceptances mailed: mid-March
> School begins: early September

*Deposit* (to hold place in class): none required.

*Deferments:* are considered on an individual basis by the Admissions Committee and may be granted for extenuating circumstances.

*Evaluation criteria*

There is a 2-part admission procedure. For the fall 2000 admission year, the class was selected based upon the following comparative evaluation:

1. *Evaluation of academic record* (weighted approximately 60 percent)

   Undergraduate cumulative GPA

   Required course GPA

   Most recent 30–45 semester credit GPA

   Test scores

2. *Evaluation of personal experience and characteristics*
   (weighted approximately 40 percent)

   Animal and veterinary work experience

   Other preparatory experience (includes extracurricular activities)

   Personal history/academic performance (summary category to include review of academic history, academic achievements, diversity of background, etc.)

   Reference letters

*2000–2001 admissions summary*

|  |  | Number of Applicants | Number of New Entrants |
|---|---|---|---|
| Resident |  | 187 | 68 |
| Nonresident |  | 1,084 | 12 |
|  | Total: | 1,271 | 80 |

## Expenses for the 2000–2001 Academic Year

*Tuition and fees*

| | |
|---|---|
| Resident | $13,542.00 |
| Nonresident | $20,404.00 |

## Dual-Degree Programs

Combined DVM–graduate degree programs are available.

# Veterinary Medical Schools in Canada

## University of Guelph

Admissions, Office of Registrarial Services
University Centre, Level 3
University of Guelph
Guelph Ontario N1G 2W1
Canada
Telephone: (519) 824-4120, ext. 6062
www.ovc.uoguelph.ca

Founded in 1862, the Ontario Veterinary College is located in Guelph about 60 miles north of Buffalo. Guelph has a similar climate to Detroit and Chicago. Surrounded by gently rolling farmland, this city of 90,000 is typical of the northeast.

The university has an enrollment of 12,220 undergraduate students, of whom 400 are veterinary students. There are also approximately 150 graduate students, 100 faculty, and 200 staff members at the veterinary college, which offers degree programs leading to a DVM, MS, PhD, Doctor of Veterinary Science (DVSc) and a Graduate Diploma. The college has 4 departments— Population Medicine, Clinical Studies, Biomedical Sciences, and Pathobiology —and a full-service teaching hospital. Funding for research comes from 2 sources: the Ontario Ministry of Agriculture, Food and Rural Affairs research contract of 4.6 million $C and external research grants and contracts of 3.9 million $C. There are also large, modern research stations for separately housing sheep, swine, and dairy and beef cattle.

### Application Information

For specific application information (availability, deadlines, fees, and VMCAS participation), please refer to the contact information listed above.

*Residency implications:* Canadian citizens or individuals who have permanent resident status of at least one year's duration who are residents of Ontario will be considered. International applicants will be considered provided the applicant does not hold Canadian citizenship or permanent resident status in Canada. There is a maximum of 5 international positions available per year.

## Prerequisites for Admission

*Course requirements and semester hours:* Students must first complete a minimum of two full-time years (four full-time semesters) of university including specific university courses. Students initially apply for admission to a science degree program. For the purpose of DVM admission, a full-time semester will include at least 5 one-semester courses. Once the prerequisite courses are completed successfully, students apply for admission to the DVM Program.

The subject matter requirements listed below must have been completed before admission to the DVM program will be considered.

*Course requirements and semesters*

| | |
|---|---|
| Biological sciences (emphasis on animal biology; one semester must be cell biology) | 3 |
| Genetics | 1 |
| Biochemistry | 1 |
| Statistics (with a university-level calculus prerequisite) | 1 |
| Humanities or social sciences* | 2 |

\* Students entering the DVM program should be able to operate across discipline boundaries recognizing the relevance of the humanities and social sciences to their career choice. In selecting these courses from among those acceptable, the prospective veterinary student should consider topics such as ethics, logic, critical thinking, determinants of human behavior, and human social interaction.

Required courses proposed to be completed at an institution other than the University of Guelph should be approved as acceptable prior to registration. Applicants are required to request approval for courses in writing. Course descriptions *must* be included with the request. Courses will *not* be acceptable if they are repeats of previously passed courses, or if they are taken at the same or a lower level in a subject area than previously passed courses in the same subject area. It is expected that the required undergraduate preparation for the DVM program will be completed in a full-time coherent academic program.

*Required undergraduate GPA:* students with a minimum A (80% — GPA 3.60) based on the average of the required courses and the last 2 semesters in full-time attendance at university may be further considered.

*Course completion deadline:* required courses must be completed by June 15 of the year of application in order to be further considered.

*Standardized examinations:* Medical College Admission Test (MCAT) is required. Test scores must be received no later than December 1 of the year of application. (Applicants unable to submit MCAT scores may submit GRE scores.)

*Additional requirements and considerations*
   Reasons for choosing a career in veterinary medicine
   Quality of preparatory academic program
   Experience and knowledge in matters relating to animals and to the veterinary medical profession
   Experience and achievement in extracurricular affairs and/or community service activities
   Communication skills
   Referees' reports

## Summary of Admission Procedure

*Timetable*
   Application deadline: October 1 for VMCAS applications; December 1 for all others
   Date interviews are held: February–June
   Date acceptances mailed: March–July
   School begins: September

*Deposit* (to hold place in class): $500.00

*2000–2001 admissions summary*

|  | Number of Applicants | Number of New Entrants |
|---|---|---|
| Residents | 550 | 100 |
| International Residents | 100 | 5 |
| Total: | 650 | 105 |

## Expenses for the 2000–2001 Academic Year

*Tuition and fees*
| Resident | $5,500.00 $C |
|---|---|
| Visa student | $38,000.00 $C |

# Université de Montréal

Service des Admissions
Université de Montréal
C.P. 6205
Succursale Centre-Ville
Montréal Québec H3C 3T5
Canada
Téléphone: (514) 343-7076
E-mail: saefmv@medvet.umontreal.ca
www.medvet.umontreal.ca

## Renseignements pour les applications/Application Information

*Formulaires disponibles dès: décembre*
*Applications available:* December

*Date limite de remise:* 1$^{er}$ mars
*Application deadline:* March 1

*Frais d'application:* 30.00 $C
*Application fee:* 30.00 $C

*Statut de résident:* Il faut être citoyen Canadien ou résident permanent pour être admissible.
*Residency implications:* Canadian citizenship or permanent residency in Canada is required.

## Prérequis/Prerequisites for Admission

DEC (Diplôme d'Etudes Collégiales) en sciences de la nature
DEC (Junior College Diploma: obtained in Quebec) majoring in nature science. (The DEC represents 2 years of post-high school studies.)

*Cours/Course requirements*

| | |
|---|---|
| Physique/Physics | 101, 201, 301–78 |
| Chimie/Chemistry | 101, 201, 202 |
| Biologie/Biology | 301, 401 |
| Mathématiques (avec calcul intégral)/ Mathematics (including calculus) | 103, 203 |

Pour être admis au programme de DMV, il faut: a) avoir satisfait les conditions ci-dessus, ou b) faire preuve d'études équivalentes.

To be considered for admission, one must: a) have completed the above requirements, or b) have completed equivalent studies.

Note: All lectures are given in French. Examinations must be written in French.

Le programme de DMV est maintenant réparti sur cinq ans.

The DMV is now a 5-year program.

*La Maîtrise de la langue française* est une condition de diplômation. Par conséquent, tout nouvel étudiant doit réussir le test de français du Ministère de l'Education ou, s'il échoue au test, réussir les cours de français prescrits par l'Université.

*Language requirements:* All students entering undergraduate degree programs must show that they have mastery of the French language in order to qualify for the degree. This graduation requirement may be met either by passing the Quebec Department of Education French test or by passing designated remedial French courses.

*Test de Français:* Le succès à ce test n'est pas obligatoire pour l'admission mais l'étudiant doit le réussir pour obtenir son diplôme.

*French test:* Success in passing this language test is not a prerequisite for admission in first year of the veterinary program, but each student must pass the test successfully to earn a diploma.

*Performance Score:* This score is obtained by comparing the student's grade in each course with the class average.

*Dossier academique avant admission:* Le candidat doit, ou bien avoir terminé, ou s'être inscrit à tous les cours prérequis au moment de l'application.

*Course completion deadline:* The applicant must be registered for or have completed all prerequisites at the time of application.

*Critères de sélection (priorité d'importance)/Additional considerations (in order of importance)*
1. Dossier académique
2. Entrevue: l'entrevue a été structurée pour évaluer la motivation, la préparation et le raisonnement des candidats.
1. Academic record
2. Interview: the interview is designed to verify the applicant's motivation, preparation, judgment, etc. The above list reflects priorities (applicants are judged first on academic merit, then test/exam results, etc.).

## Cédule du processus/Summary of Admission Procedure

*Horaire*
 Date limite de remise des formules: le 1$^{er}$ mars
 Entrevues: mi-mai
 Notification d'acceptation: fin mai, début juin
 Début de l'année scolaire: fin août

*Timetable*
 Application deadline: March 1
 Interviews: mid-May
 Notification of acceptance: end of May, early June
 Fall semester begins: end of August

*Dépôt nécessaire pour garder une place dans la classe:* aucun.
*Deposit (to hold place in class):* none required.

L'acceptation ne peut, en aucun cas, être reportée à une année subséquente.
*Deferments:* not considered.

| Critères d'évaluation/Evaluation criteria | % |
|---|---|
| Résultats scolaires/Performance score | 60 |
| Entrevue/Interview | 40 |

## Budget estimé/Estimated Expenses for the 2000–2001 Academic Year

| *Frais de scolarité:* | 55.61 \$C | par credit |
| | | (approx. 50 credits par année) |
| *Tuition and fees:* | 55.61 \$C | per credit |
| | | (approx. 50 per year) |

# University of Prince Edward Island

Registrar's Office
Atlantic Veterinary College
University of Prince Edward Island
550 University Avenue
Charlottetown PEI C1A 4P3
Canada
Telephone: (902) 566-0608
E-mail: registrar@upei.ca
www.upei.ca/~regoff/

The Atlantic Veterinary College (AVC), one of the newest colleges of veterinary medicine in North America, was completed in 1986 and is fully accredited by the American Veterinary Medical Association, the Canadian Veterinary Medical Association, and the Royal College of Veterinary Surgeons (UK).

Centrally located on Canada's eastern seaboard (650 miles northeast of Boston), the Atlantic Veterinary College makes its home in a beautiful island setting in Charlottetown, Prince Edward Island. With a population of 135,000, which jumps to over a million during the summer tourist season, the community enjoys a small-town lifestyle that boasts the amenities of larger cities, including dining and theatre. Residents also enjoy outdoor activities, such as golfing, cycling, sailing, and cross-country skiing.

The college is a completely integrated teaching, research, and service facility. The four-story complex contains the veterinary teaching hospital, diagnostic services, fish health unit, farm services, postmortem services, animal barns, laboratories, classrooms, computer and audio-visual facilities, offices, cafeteria, and study areas. The Atlantic Veterinary College also operates a nearby farm facility, a swine research facility, and a fish hatchery.

Prince Edward Island is a scenic province with a wide variety of dairy, beef, hog, sheep, horse, and fish farms. The combination and variety of animal and fish farms have allowed AVC to develop a special expertise in fish health, aquaculture, and population medicine.

## Application Information

For specific application information (availability, deadlines, fees, and VMCAS participation), please refer to the contact information listed above.

*Residency implications:* Atlantic Veterinary College contracts with New Brunswick (13), Newfoundland (2), Nova Scotia (16), and the home province P.E.I. (10). International students are admitted on a noncontract basis (19).

**Prerequisites for Admission**

The preveterinary program leading to admission at the Atlantic Veterinary College will normally take 2 years to complete.

*Course requirements*
The equivalent of 20 one-semester courses are required, including:
    Mathematics, 2 courses, including statistics
    Biology, 4 courses, including genetics and microbiology
    Chemistry, 3 courses, including organic chemistry
    Physics, 1 course
    English, 2 courses, one of which must be a course in English composition
    Humanities and social sciences, 3 courses
    Electives, 5 courses from any discipline
    (Science courses will normally have a laboratory component.)

*Required undergraduate GPA:* no minimum stated; mean cumulative GPA of most recent entering class is 3.14 on a 4.00 scale.

*AP credit policy:* not accepted.

*Course completion deadline:* June 1 of the year of application.

*Standardized examinations:* Graduate Record Examination (GRE) (for non-Canadian applicants only). If a student's native language or language of prior education is not English, then the student will be required to pass one of the following: TOEFL, MELAB, IELB, or CanTest.

*Additional requirements and considerations*
    Veterinary-related experience: at least two 40-hour experiences with veterinarians in practice, government, industry, or in a research environment at an academic institution are required. One of these experiences must involve clinical practice in the field. If an applicant selects 2 clinical experiences, he or she cannot be in the same field or under the supervision of the same veterinarian.
    Veterinary evaluations
    Interview
    Essay
    Additional academic achievement

## Summary of Admission Procedure

*Timetable*

Application deadline: October 1 for VMCAS applications; December 1 for all others

Date interviews are held: March–April

Date acceptances mailed: April

School begins: late August-early September; registration, early September

*Deposit* (to hold place in class): 500.00 $C

*Deferments:* are considered for extenuating circumstances.

*Evaluation criteria*

Academic credentials and animal work experience are objectively evaluated by the Registrar's Office. Other criteria and activities are subjectively evaluated by the admissions committee through an interview process.

|                                    | % weight |
| ---------------------------------- | -------- |
| Grades                             | 50       |
| Additional academic achievement    | 5        |
| Veterinary experience, interview   | 35       |
| Essay                              | 10       |

*2000-2001 admissions summary*

|              | Number of Applicants | Number of New Entrants |
| ------------ | -------------------- | ---------------------- |
| In-province  | 27                   | 10                     |
| Contract*    | 99                   | 31                     |
| International | 407                 | 19                     |
| Total:       | 533                  | 60                     |

## Expenses for the 2000-2001 Academic Year

*Tuition and fees*

|                        |               |
| ---------------------- | ------------- |
| Resident               | 6,770.00 $C   |
| Contract student*      | 6,770.00 $C   |
| International student  | 39,200.00 $C  |

\* For further information, see the listing of contracting states and provinces.

# University of Saskatchewan

Admissions Office
Western College of Veterinary Medicine
52 Campus Drive
University of Saskatchewan
Saskatoon Saskatchewan S7N 5B4
Canada
Telephone: (306) 966-7454
www.usask.ca/wcvm

The Western College of Veterinary Medicine is located in the city of Saskatoon, which has a population of about 180,000 and is the major urban center in central Saskatchewan. The city is also the major commercial center for central and northern Saskatchewan and is served by 2 national airlines with direct connections to all major centers in Canada. Summers are short and cool; winters are long and cold.

The Western College of Veterinary Medicine is one of the few veterinary colleges where all health sciences and agriculture are offered on the same campus. The college is devoted to undergraduate education and has a reputation in Canada and in the northwestern United States for educating veterinarians who are well-rounded in general veterinary medicine and have good practical backgrounds. It has one of the best field-service caseloads in North America.

## Application Information

For specific application information (availability, deadlines, fees, and VMCAS participation), please refer to the contact information listed above.

*Residency implications:* students are selected for quota positions from Alberta, British Columbia, Manitoba, Saskatchewan, and the Yukon Territory. Occasional positions are available to other Canadian residents. Special consideration is given to self-identified individuals of aboriginal origin. Residents of foreign countries where veterinary schools exist are not considered.

## Prerequisites for Admission

*Course requirements and semester hours*

| | |
|---|---|
| English | 6 |
| Physics | 6 |
| Biology | 6 |
| Genetics | 3 |
| Introductory chemistry | 6 |
| Organic chemistry | 3 |
| Mathematics or statistics | 6 |
| Biochemistry | 6 |
| Microbiology | 3 |
| Electives | 15 |

*Required undergraduate GPA:* a minimum cumulative average of 70% is required.

*Course completion deadline:* prerequisite courses must be completed by the time of entry into the program.

*Standardized examinations:* none required.

*Additional requirements and considerations*
Animal/veterinary work experience, motivation, and knowledge
Maturity
Leadership
Communication skills

## Summary of Admission Procedure

*Timetable*
Application deadline: January 3
Date interviews are held: May–June
Date acceptances mailed: on or before July 1
School begins: late August

*Deposit* (to hold place in class): none required.

*Deferments:* not considered.

*Evaluation criteria*

The 3-part admission procedure consists of an assessment of academic ability, a personal interview, and an overall assessment of the application file.

|  | *% weight* |
|---|---|
| Grades | 60 |
| Interview* | 30 |
| Judgment | 10 |

\* Interview selection is based entirely on academic performance.

*2000-2001 admissions summary*

|  | *Number of Applicants* | *Number of New Entrants* |
|---|---|---|
| Resident | 50 | 20 |
| Contract† | 262 | 50 |
| Nonresident | 3 | 0 |
| Total: | 315 | 70 |

## Expenses for the 2000-2001 Academic Year

*Tuition and fees*

|  |  |
|---|---|
| Resident | 5,810.00 $C |
| Nonresident |  |
| Contract student† | 5,810.00 $C |
| Other nonresident-Canadian | 5,810.00 $C |

† For further information, see the listing of contracting states and provinces.

# Policies on Advanced Standing

Transfers are permitted to most colleges of veterinary medicine in the United States under specified conditions. Typical requirements include a vacancy in the class, completion of all prerequisite requirements, and compatible curricula. Following is a listing of schools and some of the conditions under which they will consider a transfer from another veterinary college with advanced standing. More detailed information may be obtained by writing to the individual schools in which you have an interest.

## UNITED STATES

### University of California

1. An opening must exist in the second- or third-year class.
2. The applicant must have completed equivalent coursework to that of students in the class to which that person seeks admission.
3. The applicant must meet the minimum academic requirements for admission as stated in the Guide for Prospective Students.
4. Priority is given to California residents. It is usually not possible to determine if a position will be available until after July 1 in any given year.

### Colorado State University

Advanced standing will be considered on an individual basis subject to the following provisions:

1. An open position must be available within the applicable tuition classification category for an additional student.
2. The applicant must meet all prerequisites for admission to the program as a first-year student and possess qualifications that are competitive with currently enrolled students.
3. The applicant must have completed at least one full academic year at the institution in which currently enrolled and have achieved a cumulative GPA of 3.00 or better (of 4.00) and be in good academic standing. Transfer credit will not be allowed for any course receiving a grade of less than 2.00 (of 4.00).
4. If the applicant is acceptable to the Admissions Committee and a position is available, placement will be offered in the year and term of the curriculum deemed appropriate after analysis of equivalency of the required courses.
5. Applicant must be enrolled in an AVMA accredited college.

Students attending non-AVMA accredited institutions must apply for admission to the first-year class through the regular admissions process.

## University of Florida

1. An opening must exist in the second- or third-year class.
2. Students with advanced standing are rarely considered for admission to second- or third-year classes on the basis of exceptional personal circumstances.
3. Student must be enrolled in an AVMA accredited college.
4. Student must meet all prerequisites for admission as a first-year student (including GRE scores).
5. The curricula of the two schools must be sufficiently alike to allow a student to enter without deficiencies in academic background.
6. Applicant must *not* have been denied admission to the University of Florida College of Veterinary Medicine as a first-year student.
7. Applicants must have a letter approving transfer from their dean or associate dean.

## University of Georgia

1. Must be a resident of the United States, with priority given to Georgia residents, followed by contract state residents, then all other citizens.
2. Applicants will be considered for entry in the second or third year.
3. Applications must include a letter of support written by a senior administrator of the school in which the applicant is currently enrolled.
4. All selection criteria for regular applicants apply to transfer applicants.
5. No individual is eligible for transfer who has been dismissed or is on probation at any other school or college for deficiency in scholarship or because of misconduct.

## University of Illinois

1. Requests for transfer are considered on a case-by-case basis to maintain class size.
2. All prerequisite science courses must be completed prior to the request for transfer.
3. Minimum grade requirements include:
   cumulative and science GPAs of 2.75 on a 4.00 scale;
   semester GPA of 2.25 on a 4.00 scale for each semester of veterinary medical coursework completed (all undergraduate and current veterinary school);
   courses must be completed with a grade of C- or better (2.00 = C).

4. Student must complete the same preveterinary coursework as required for all students accepted to the program.
5. Student must be in good academic standing.
6. To request transfer consideration, student must submit a letter explaining the reasons for transfer, official transcripts from all universities/colleges attended, description of all veterinary coursework completed to date, and a letter from the dean of the current school certifying the applicant's academic standing.

### Iowa State University

1. The applicant must have had essentially the same preveterinary coursework as required of Iowa State students and must have met the minimum qualifications of those admitted to the College of Veterinary Medicine.
2. The applicant must have completed the equivalent of all courses required of Iowa State University veterinary students beginning the academic term the applicant seeks to enter. Only credits earned at an AVMA accredited college of veterinary medicine will be considered for credit.
3. The applicant must have been in good standing throughout his or her entire period of enrollment in the school(s) of veterinary medicine in which the student is, or has been, enrolled. A letter to that effect from the dean(s) of the school(s) is required.
4. Space must be available.

### Kansas State University

Acceptance of students for advanced standing is on recommendation of the Admissions Committee on a space-available basis.

### Louisiana State University

Applicants must have successfully completed all previous professional courses in an AVMA accredited college or school of veterinary medicine. The request for transfer and supporting documents are reviewed by the Committee on Admissions. After review the committee forwards a recommendation to the dean for approval or denial of the transfer request.

### Michigan State University

1. Admission consideration is offered only to those current matriculants in professional veterinary curricula who believe that there are extenuating circumstances that would precipitate significant undue hardship if they continue at their current institution.

2. Applicants must also demonstrate quality academic performance throughout their professional school enrollment.
3. The curricula of the two schools must be sufficiently alike to allow a student to enter the second-year class without deficiencies in academic background.
4. All selection criteria for regular applicants apply to transfer applicants.
5. Priority is given to Michigan residents.
6. AVMA accreditation of current school is considered.

**University of Minnesota**

1. Transfers are not allowed to any specific requested year or semester. The committee will place each applicant in the year or semester of the curriculum deemed appropriate after analysis of equivalency of the required courses involved.
2. No academic work or standing will be accepted from DVM curricula other than those deemed accredited ("AVMA accredited") or approved ("AVMA approved") by the American Veterinary Medical Association.
3. All applicants must be U.S. citizens, be holders of permanent resident alien visas, or have achieved landed immigrant status.
4. All applicants are required to have finished at least one full academic year at the institution from which transfer is requested and must be in good academic standing at the time of discontinuance according to written verification from the institution.
5. All applicants must document that not more than two calendar years have elapsed between discontinuance and application to our DVM program.
6. All applicants must have achieved a cumulative GPA of 3.00 (of 4.00) for the required courses at the initial institution.
7. All applicants must present suitable transcripts and course summary descriptions of all courses taken. These must be carried to the appropriate course coordinator in our curriculum, and each coordinator must certify in writing that the transfer courses satisfy our curricular specifications according to comparative criteria determined by each coordinator in discussion with the petitioner. The applicant is responsible for preparing a standard University of Minnesota Petition Form, obtaining the course instructor's dated signature, and returning it to the Office for Student Affairs and Admission. If equivalency is not certified, the course must be taken in our curriculum prior to the transfer to a specific veterinary class year.

## Mississippi State University

A limited number of transfer students are accepted in order to maintain a stable class size. Transfer positions are filled on a competitive basis.

1. Applicants must attend an interview at the College of Veterinary Medicine to be eligible for admission.
2. Applicants must submit complete transcripts of all DVM coursework.
3. Transfers are limited to the first two years of the curriculum. No student can transfer into the curriculum beyond the start of the third year of the professional program.
4. Candidates must demonstrate quality academic performance and professional behavior to be considered for transfer. Transfer applicants who have failed one or more courses at another college of veterinary medicine will not be considered for admission. Transfer applicants who have been dismissed for academic or other reasons from any other college of veterinary medicine will not be considered for admission.
5. To initiate transfer, candidates must submit a formal letter of intent, stating reasons for transfer, and an official transcript from their professional program.

## University of Missouri

1. Must be a vacancy in the class.
2. Will consider students who are U.S. citizens or holders of permanent alien visas and who have finished at least two years in a college of veterinary medicine that is AVMA accredited.
3. Students must be in good academic standing, and a letter of reference from the dean's office of the present college is required.

## North Carolina State University

1. Must be a vacancy in the class.
2. Consideration by the Admission Committee on an individual basis.
3. Curricula must be compatible.
4. Support letter required from the dean's office.
5. Letter of recommendation from a faculty member at the original college.
6. Only accept transfers from AVMA accredited colleges.
7. At least 50% of DVM credit hours should be completed at North Carolina State in order to earn a North Carolina State degree.

## Ohio State University

1. An opening must exist.
2. Student must be enrolled in an AVMA accredited college.

3. The curricula of the two schools must be sufficiently alike to allow the student to enter a class without deficiencies in his or her academic background.
4. Student must be in good academic standing in present college and have a supporting letter from the Dean of Student and Academic Affairs to this effect.
5. Each request for transfer is considered on an individual basis, taking into account personal hardship, family situations, etc.
6. Must meet same prerequisite requirements as first-year applicants.

## Oklahoma State University

1. A student will normally enter at the beginning of the fall semester, second year, regardless of his/her standing at the school from which he/she is transferring.
2. A student may be accepted only if a vacancy exists in the second-year class, fall semester.
3. Preference will be given to students from schools/colleges with AVMA accreditation.
4. Application deadline is April 15, with all requirements having been met prior to entry date.
5. Applications accepted only from students from institutions that are accredited by an authentic accrediting agency.

## Oregon State University

Admission of students with advanced standing is considered only in very specific and unique circumstances, and each case is considered on an individual basis.

## University of Pennsylvania

1. An opening must exist.
2. Admission with Advanced Standing (AAS) is considered only from institutions that are accredited by the AVMA.
3. Student must initiate the process at his/her own institution. The Dean of Student Affairs at the college from which the student wants to transfer must understand the student's need for AAS and endorse it. The usual reasons endorsed are either medical or the desire to move nearer one's spouse.
4. If the Dean of Student Affairs approves, student must send detailed description of all coursework taken to date and simultaneously submit an application to the University of Pennsylvania's Admissions Committee. If the Admissions Committee accepts the credentials, it will compare coursework

with that of the University of Pennsylvania and determine where in the curriculum the student might be placed.

5. If all criteria are met and space is available, AAS may be granted.
6. University of Pennsylvania cannot award a degree to a student who has completed less than 50% of graduation credits at Penn.

## Purdue University

1. Must be a vacancy in the class.
2. Curricula must be compatible.
3. Must be in good academic standing at present college.
4. Must have an acceptable undergraduate record as determined by the Admissions Committee.
5. Admission limited to the first or second year of the program.

## University of Tennessee

Admission of students with advanced standing may be considered for unique circumstances on a case-by-case basis. Space must be available in the class and the professional curricula must reasonably match between the schools. The Admissions Committee will review applicants' credentials and interview those determined to best meet admission criteria. Admission is usually limited to the second semester of the first year of the professional curriculum. Students must be in good standing at their present college.

## Texas A & M University

Students requesting advanced standing must meet the following requirements:

1. Must have completed all previous professional veterinary courses in an AVMA accredited college of veterinary medicine.
2. Must have successfully completed the academic term preceding the semester into which student requests admission.
3. Must comply with all requirements for transfer into the university as described in the current catalog.
4. May request transfer only into the second through seventh semesters of the professional curriculum.
5. At the time of matriculation the student must certify by letter that he/she has not been convicted of crimes in the period from first enrollment in the college of veterinary medicine from which the student desires transfer until date of matriculation at Texas A&M University.
6. To request transfer consideration, the student must:

submit a letter explaining the reason(s) for requesting transfer, desired date of transfer, and class and semester of curriculum into which transfer is requested; and provide a letter of character and academic reference (including class ranking) from the dean of the college from which student desires the transfer; two letters of reference from former instructors who are members of the faculty of the college from which student desires the transfer; and official copies of all academic transcripts.

## Tufts University

Applicants from other veterinary schools are considered. Students with advanced standing are admitted if and when space becomes available in the second- or third-year class. The application deadline is June 1 for the following September.

## Virginia Polytechnic Institute and State University

1. Applicants may be a Virginia or Maryland resident or a nonresident enrolled in another veterinary school.
2. Advanced standing is allowed only if a vacancy exists. Class size cannot exceed 90 students. Must start at the beginning of second or third year.
3. Must have a 3.00 GPA in veterinary school attended.
4. Must submit transcripts from all colleges attended and meet minimum GPA requirements for all college work.
5. Must have completed the same preprofessional courses required for first-year admission with a grade of C- or higher.
6. Must have prevet credentials that would have resulted in an offer of admission or placement on the alternate list for a position in the class/year being requested.
7. Letters from current dean and two faculty members are required.
8. Petition for advanced standing, with reasons for same, must be received by May 1 of the year in which transfer occurs.

## Washington State University

Admission of students with advanced standing is effected only in very specific and unique circumstances, and each case is considered on an individual basis.

## University of Wisconsin

Requests will be evaluated using the same selection criteria established for applicants to the first-year class and will be considered under the following circumstances:

1. Applicant will be considered for admission only if there is space available in the class into which he/she wishes to enter.
2. The applicant must have attended an AVMA accredited college of veterinary medicine.
3. Applicant must have passed all professional courses and attained the minimum cumulative GPA required for promotion of students.
4. Wisconsin residents will be given first consideration for admission if the above criteria have been met.

## CANADA

### University of Guelph

Admission with advanced standing from other veterinary schools will be considered provided a vacancy exists and the applicant can fulfill the residence requirements and has a satisfactory academic record. The occurrence of vacancies is extremely rare.

### University of Prince Edward Island

Applicants who have completed all or portions of a veterinary medical program may apply for advanced standing to the second year of the DVM program. Applicants for advanced standing must present evidence of educational accomplishments and may be required to satisfactorily pass examinations in all of the courses for which they desire credit. Students admitted with advanced standing must begin the college year in September.

The candidate must file a formal application and may be interviewed by the Admissions Committee and possibly other faculty. Places for admission to the college with advanced standing are limited and depend on vacancies.

It is imperative that the Admissions Committee have detailed and translated summaries of veterinary medical academic programs and accomplishments for those seeking advanced placement from schools in foreign countries. Advanced-standing applications should be on file and completed as early as possible and no later than January 1.

### University of Saskatchewan

1. Must have a vacancy.
2. Curricula must be compatible.
3. Residency requirements apply.
4. There is no admission beyond the second year.
5. GRE is required.
6. TOEFL is required if first language is not English.

# Application and Enrollment Data

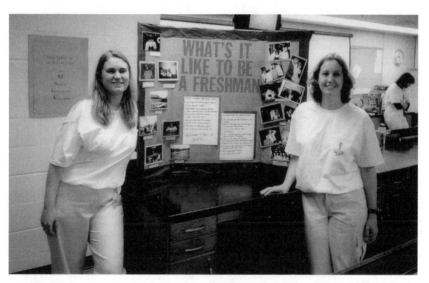

Many colleges of veterinary medicine hold open houses — a great way to help potential students learn the ropes. Photo courtesy of Auburn University, College of Veterinary Medicine.

## Table 1
## Applications and Applicants to Colleges of Veterinary Medicine, 1977–99

| Year | Number of Colleges | First Year Positions | Number of Applications | Applications per Position | Applicants |
|------|------|------|------|------|------|
| 1977 | 22 | 1,973 | 10,704 | 5.43 | — |
| 1978 | 22 | 2,086 | 9,467 | 4.54 | — |
| 1979 | 24 | 2,296 | 10,120 | 4.41 | — |
| 1980 | 25 | 2,213 | 9,525 | 4.30 | 7,286 |
| 1981 | 26 | 2,220 | 8,367 | 3.65 | 6,373 |
| 1982 | 26 | 2,231 | 8,262 | 3.70 | 6,182 |
| 1983* | 27 | 2,306 | 8,074 | 3.50 | 5,805 |
| 1984 | 27 | 2,300 | 8,291 | 3.60 | 5,503 |
| 1985 | 27 | 2,282 | 7,953 | 3.49 | 4,961 |
| 1986 | 27 | 2,277 | 7,719 | 3.39 | 4,751 |
| 1987 | 27 | 2,199 | 7,729 | 3.51 | 4,432 |
| 1988 | 27 | 2,195 | 7,422 | 3.38 | 4,200 |
| 1989 | 27 | 2,189 | 7,098 | 3.24 | 3,922 |
| 1990 | 27 | 2,191 | 7,218 | 3.29 | 3,955 |
| 1991 | 27 | 2,172 | 7,848 | 3.61 | 4,296 |
| 1992 | 27 | 2,317 | 8,737 | 3.77 | 4,709 |
| 1993 | 27 | 2,309 | 9,939 | 4.30 | 4,957 |
| 1994 | 27 | 2,314 | 10,961 | 4.74 | 5,428 |
| 1995 | 27 | 2,290 | 12,499 | 5.46 | 6,634 |
| 1996† | 27 | 2,322 | 22,578 | 9.72 | 6,424 |
| 1997 | 27 | 2,302 | 23,595 | 10.25 | 6,630 |
| 1998 | 27 | 2,330 | 27,312 | 11.72 | 6,783 |
| 1999 | 27 | 2,301 | 24,448 | 10.62 | 6,695 |

\* Data for 1983 may be inconsistent due to incomplete reporting from two colleges.
† Year 1 of VMCAS operations

## Table 2
## Acceptance of First-Time and Repeat Applicants, 1995–99

| Applicants | 1995 | | | 1996 | | |
|------|------|------|------|------|------|------|
| | Total Number | Number Accepted | Percent Accepted | Total Number | Number Accepted | Percent Accepted |
| First-time | 4,879 | 1,714 | 35.1 | 4,740 | 1,740 | 36.7 |
| Repeat | 1,755 | 566 | 32.3 | 1,684 | 553 | 32.8 |
| Total | 6,634 | 2,280 | 34.4 | 6,424 | 2,293 | 35.7 |

| Applicants per Position | Percentage Accepted* | Applications per Applicant | Repeat Applicants | New Applicants |
|---|---|---|---|---|
| – | – | – | – | – |
| – | – | – | – | – |
| – | – | – | – | – |
| 3.29 | 30.40 | 1.31 | – | – |
| 2.87 | 34.80 | 1.31 | – | – |
| 2.77 | 36.10 | 1.34 | – | – |
| 2.52 | 39.80 | 1.39 | 2,121 | 3,684 |
| 2.39 | 41.80 | 1.51 | 1,842 | 3,661 |
| 2.17 | 46.00 | 1.60 | 1,660 | 3,301 |
| 2.09 | 47.93 | 1.62 | 1,394 | 3,357 |
| 2.02 | 49.62 | 1.74 | 1,252 | 3,180 |
| 1.91 | 52.26 | 1.77 | 1,095 | 3,105 |
| 1.79 | 55.81 | 1.81 | 984 | 2,938 |
| 1.81 | 55.40 | 1.83 | 862 | 3,093 |
| 1.98 | 50.56 | 1.83 | 861 | 3,435 |
| 2.03 | 49.20 | 1.86 | 960 | 3,749 |
| 2.15 | 46.58 | 2.01 | 1,117 | 3,840 |
| 2.35 | 42.63 | 2.02 | 1,380 | 4,048 |
| 2.89 | 34.40 | 1.88 | 1,755 | 4,879 |
| 2.77 | 35.70 | 3.51 | 1,684 | 4,740 |
| 2.88 | 33.29 | 3.56 | 1,930 | 4,700 |
| 2.91 | 32.27 | 4.03 | 2,306 | 4,477 |
| 2.91 | 32.83 | 3.65 | 2,366 | 4,329 |

| 1997 | | | 1998 | | | 1999 | | |
|---|---|---|---|---|---|---|---|---|
| Total Number | Number Accepted | Percent Accepted | Total Number | Number Accepted | Percent Accepted | Total Number | Number Accepted | Percent Accepted |
| 4,700 | 1,654 | 35.19 | 4,477 | 1,528 | 34.13 | 4,329 | 1,521 | 35.14 |
| 1,930 | 553 | 28.65 | 2,306 | 661 | 28.66 | 2,366 | 677 | 28.61 |
| 6,630 | 2,207 | 33.29 | 6,783 | 2,189 | 32.27 | 6,695 | 2,198 | 32.83 |

## Table 3

**Applications per Position in Entering Class in U.S. Colleges of Veterinary Medicine, 1995-99**

| College | 1995 | | | 1996 | | |
|---------|------|------|------|------|------|------|
| | A | P | A/P | A | P | A/P |
| Auburn Univ | 446 | 92 | 4.85 | 917 | 90 | 10.19 |
| Univ of California | 552 | 108 | 5.11 | 736 | 109 | 6.75 |
| Colorado State | 764 | 132 | 5.79 | 746 | 134 | 5.57 |
| Cornell Univ | 622 | 82 | 7.59 | 732 | 80 | 9.15 |
| Univ of Florida | 487 | 80 | 6.09 | 766 | 80 | 9.58 |
| Univ of Georgia | 431 | 87 | 4.95 | 763 | 92 | 8.29 |
| Univ of Illinois | 379 | 87 | 4.36 | 736 | 87 | 8.46 |
| Iowa State | 690 | 100 | 6.90 | 1,773 | 102 | 17.38 |
| Kansas State | 341 | 107 | 3.19 | 559 | 107 | 5.22 |
| Louisiana State | 371 | 80 | 4.64 | 1,075 | 80 | 13.44 |
| Michigan State | 554 | 100 | 5.54 | 1,375 | 111 | 12.39 |
| Univ of Minnesota | 489 | 76 | 6.43 | 1,168 | 76 | 15.37 |
| Mississippi State | 167 | 49 | 3.41 | 340 | 49 | 6.94 |
| Univ of Missouri | 295 | 64 | 4.61 | 254 | 64 | 3.97 |
| North Carolina State | 500 | 78 | 6.41 | 1,021 | 72 | 14.18 |
| Ohio State | 423 | 133 | 3.18 | 478 | 133 | 3.59 |
| Oklahoma State | 411 | 71 | 5.79 | 682 | 74 | 9.22 |
| Oregon State | 324 | 36 | 9.00 | 892 | 36 | 24.78 |
| Univ of Pennsylvania | 744 | 109 | 6.83 | 1,307 | 105 | 12.45 |
| Purdue Univ | 506 | 69 | 7.33 | 925 | 65 | 14.23 |
| Univ of Tennessee | 334 | 63 | 5.30 | 566 | 68 | 8.32 |
| Texas A&M | 431 | 128 | 3.37 | 591 | 128 | 4.62 |
| Tufts Univ | 685 | 75 | 9.13 | 672 | 79 | 8.51 |
| Tuskegee Univ | 208 | 62 | 3.35 | 267 | 61 | 4.38 |
| VA-MD Regional | 249 | 80 | 3.11 | 560 | 90 | 6.22 |
| Washington State | 502 | 62 | 8.10 | 1,202 | 70 | 17.17 |
| Univ of Wisconsin | 594 | 80 | 7.43 | 1,475 | 80 | 18.44 |
| Total | 12,499 | 2,290 | 5.46 | 22,578 | 2,322 | 9.72 |

A = Applications

P = Positions in entering class as reported in this survey

A/P = Applications received per position

| 1997 | | | 1998 | | | 1999 | | |
|---|---|---|---|---|---|---|---|---|
| A | P | A/P | A | P | A/P | A | P | A/P |
| 877 | 90 | 9.74 | 934 | 90 | 10.38 | 819 | 90 | 9.10 |
| 814 | 108 | 7.54 | 1,134 | 109 | 10.40 | 1,058 | 108 | 9.80 |
| 758 | 134 | 5.66 | 804 | 134 | 6.00 | 845 | 133 | 6.35 |
| 1,178 | 82 | 14.37 | 1,517 | 82 | 18.50 | 1,239 | 81 | 15.30 |
| 745 | 80 | 9.31 | 853 | 80 | 10.66 | 812 | 80 | 10.15 |
| 681 | 80 | 8.51 | 831 | 92 | 9.03 | 820 | 81 | 10.12 |
| 481 | 101 | 4.76 | 1,264 | 101 | 12.51 | 1,073 | 100 | 10.73 |
| 1,665 | 100 | 16.65 | 1,787 | 102 | 17.52 | 1,126 | 100 | 11.26 |
| 737 | 100 | 7.37 | 1,278 | 100 | 12.78 | 728 | 100 | 7.28 |
| 1,073 | 80 | 13.41 | 1,284 | 80 | 16.05 | 1,144 | 80 | 14.30 |
| 1,218 | 100 | 12.18 | 1,324 | 111 | 11.93 | 1,317 | 101 | 13.04 |
| 1,174 | 76 | 15.45 | 1,155 | 76 | 15.20 | 1,036 | 76 | 13.63 |
| 336 | 49 | 6.86 | 415 | 49 | 8.47 | 466 | 49 | 9.51 |
| 232 | 64 | 3.63 | 238 | 64 | 3.72 | 221 | 64 | 3.45 |
| 1,084 | 72 | 15.06 | 1,162 | 72 | 16.14 | 1,150 | 72 | 15.97 |
| 1,122 | 135 | 8.31 | 1,048 | 133 | 7.88 | 1,012 | 133 | 7.61 |
| 638 | 70 | 9.11 | 635 | 74 | 8.58 | 470 | 74 | 6.35 |
| 964 | 36 | 26.78 | 1,167 | 36 | 32.42 | 986 | 37 | 26.65 |
| 1,203 | 110 | 10.94 | 1,354 | 110 | 12.31 | 1,378 | 107 | 12.88 |
| 852 | 60 | 14.20 | 1,000 | 60 | 16.67 | 947 | 60 | 15.78 |
| 589 | 68 | 8.66 | 606 | 68 | 8.91 | 463 | 68 | 6.81 |
| 1,010 | 128 | 7.89 | 1,082 | 128 | 8.45 | 955 | 128 | 7.46 |
| 714 | 79 | 9.04 | 698 | 79 | 8.84 | 759 | 79 | 9.61 |
| 298 | 60 | 4.97 | 263 | 60 | 4.38 | 216 | 60 | 3.60 |
| 750 | 90 | 8.33 | 951 | 90 | 10.57 | 992 | 90 | 11.02 |
| 1,105 | 70 | 15.79 | 1,160 | 70 | 16.57 | 1,090 | 70 | 15.57 |
| 1,297 | 80 | 16.21 | 1,368 | 80 | 17.10 | 1,326 | 80 | 16.58 |
| 23,595 | 2,302 | 10.25 | 27,312 | 2,330 | 11.72 | 24,448 | 2,301 | 10.62 |

## Table 4
## Applicants to U.S. Colleges of Veterinary Medicine by Residence, 1989-99

| Residence | 1989 | 1990 | 1991 | 1992 | 1993 | 1994 |
|---|---|---|---|---|---|---|
| Alabama | 117 | 122 | 116 | 124 | 129 | 135 |
| Alaska | 13 | 11 | 14 | 17 | 15 | 11 |
| Arizona | 30 | 35 | 51 | 50 | 59 | 70 |
| Arkansas | 26 | 25 | 30 | 30 | 44 | 30 |
| California | 377 | 353 | 409 | 439 | 386 | 434 |
| Colorado | 142 | 143 | 174 | 203 | 230 | 274 |
| Connecticut | 54 | 47 | 50 | 24 | 46 | 57 |
| Delaware | 7 | 7 | 13 | 9 | 13 | 9 |
| Dist. of Col. | — | 4 | — | 1 | — | 5 |
| Florida | 165 | 144 | 143 | 176 | 188 | 197 |
| Georgia | 109 | 90 | 112 | 136 | 134 | 153 |
| Hawaii | 17 | 21 | 16 | 16 | 18 | 18 |
| Idaho | 16 | 19 | 27 | 31 | 31 | 38 |
| Illinois | 149 | 184 | 185 | 209 | 210 | 233 |
| Indiana | 75 | 74 | 91 | 117 | 111 | 116 |
| Iowa | 83 | 110 | 135 | 81 | 130 | 95 |
| Kansas | 75 | 53 | 66 | 90 | 88 | 99 |
| Kentucky | 44 | 53 | 71 | 80 | 97 | 93 |
| Louisiana | 60 | 66 | 81 | 83 | 93 | 99 |
| Maine | 12 | 14 | 16 | 11 | 16 | 24 |
| Maryland | 90 | 87 | 87 | 105 | 107 | 156 |
| Massachusetts | 121 | 95 | 102 | 106 | 100 | 153 |
| Michigan | 151 | 165 | 149 | 181 | 140 | 175 |
| Minnesota | 67 | 79 | 91 | 96 | 112 | 104 |
| Mississippi | 67 | 61 | 60 | 55 | 37 | 43 |
| Missouri | 77 | 69 | 78 | 96 | 91 | 121 |
| Montana | 25 | 20 | 24 | 24 | 18 | 31 |
| Nebraska | 27 | 33 | 41 | 45 | 48 | 61 |
| Nevada | 25 | 10 | 14 | 13 | 16 | 22 |
| New Hampshire | 11 | 12 | 15 | 24 | 22 | 20 |
| New Jersey | 99 | 103 | 106 | 126 | 94 | 97 |

Due to multiple sources of data for each applicant, the total count per state may exceed the total number of applicants.

| 1995 | 1996 | 1997 | 1998 | 1999 | % Change 1989-99 | % Change 1998-99 |
|------|------|------|------|------|------|------|
| 153 | 134 | 152 | 169 | 153 | 30.8 | -9.5 |
| 11 | 26 | 5 | 13 | 7 | -46.2 | -46.2 |
| 101 | 83 | 70 | 63 | 74 | 146.7 | 17.5 |
| 43 | 41 | 30 | 53 | 36 | 38.5 | -32.1 |
| 545 | 495 | 524 | 553 | 538 | 42.7 | -2.7 |
| 300 | 297 | 328 | 337 | 350 | 146.5 | 3.9 |
| 94 | 61 | 61 | 48 | 50 | -7.4 | 4.2 |
| 13 | 16 | 13 | 13 | 18 | 157.1 | 38.5 |
| 7 | 7 | 4 | 5 | 1 | — | -80.0 |
| 239 | 258 | 289 | 276 | 265 | 60.6 | -4.0 |
| 194 | 199 | 207 | 214 | 239 | 119.3 | 11.7 |
| 30 | 19 | 27 | 24 | 24 | 41.2 | — |
| 46 | 33 | 42 | 43 | 41 | 156.3 | -4.7 |
| 261 | 238 | 221 | 255 | 263 | 76.5 | 3.1 |
| 133 | 125 | 119 | 122 | 126 | 68.0 | 3.3 |
| 110 | 154 | 177 | 156 | 128 | 54.2 | -17.9 |
| 91 | 115 | 121 | 97 | 118 | 57.3 | 21.6 |
| 97 | 92 | 122 | 113 | 102 | 131.8 | -9.7 |
| 114 | 129 | 197 | 201 | 202 | 236.7 | 0.5 |
| 54 | 22 | 20 | 15 | 11 | -8.3 | -26.7 |
| 119 | 119 | 130 | 132 | 144 | 60.0 | 9.1 |
| 220 | 178 | 182 | 171 | 182 | 50.4 | 6.4 |
| 209 | 230 | 249 | 259 | 226 | 49.7 | -12.7 |
| 177 | 135 | 136 | 145 | 137 | 104.5 | -5.5 |
| 50 | 57 | 91 | 83 | 79 | 17.9 | -4.8 |
| 132 | 129 | 143 | 146 | 158 | 105.2 | 8.2 |
| 32 | 32 | 34 | 45 | 39 | 56.0 | -13.3 |
| 60 | 66 | 85 | 70 | 65 | 140.7 | -7.1 |
| 22 | 28 | 29 | 20 | 15 | -40.0 | -25.0 |
| 29 | 30 | 23 | 33 | 27 | 145.5 | -18.2 |
| 112 | 114 | 136 | 121 | 123 | 24.2 | 1.7 |

## Table 4 (cont.)

| State | 1989 | 1990 | 1991 | 1992 | 1993 | 1994 |
|---|---|---|---|---|---|---|
| New Mexico | 26 | 21 | 34 | 33 | 33 | 40 |
| New York | 244 | 267 | 227 | 268 | 221 | 258 |
| North Carolina | 115 | 97 | 109 | 115 | 157 | 196 |
| North Dakota | 11 | 11 | 13 | 13 | 17 | 23 |
| Ohio | 158 | 198 | 178 | 186 | 187 | 199 |
| Oklahoma | 59 | 74 | 52 | 81 | 81 | 107 |
| Oregon | 50 | 45 | 55 | 67 | 63 | 41 |
| Pennsylvania | 153 | 155 | 176 | 179 | 187 | 186 |
| Puerto Rico | 24 | 35 | 43 | 48 | 37 | 47 |
| Rhode Island | 7 | 13 | 10 | 12 | 13 | 23 |
| South Carolina | 35 | 35 | 26 | 30 | 51 | 57 |
| South Dakota | 4 | 10 | 9 | 12 | 4 | 5 |
| Tennessee | 74 | 65 | 73 | 78 | 93 | 112 |
| Texas | 229 | 252 | 293 | 282 | 312 | 347 |
| Utah | 16 | 17 | 17 | 32 | 29 | 32 |
| Vermont | 17 | 13 | 5 | 11 | 16 | 16 |
| Virginia | 120 | 109 | 110 | 128 | 117 | 155 |
| Virgin Islands | — | 1 | — | 1 | 2 | 3 |
| Washington | 92 | 64 | 92 | 107 | 149 | 138 |
| West Virginia | 12 | 18 | 18 | 25 | 25 | 24 |
| Wisconsin | 104 | 96 | 126 | 130 | 134 | 172 |
| Wyoming | 9 | 11 | 14 | 15 | 16 | 19 |
| UNITED STATES | 3,890 | 3,916 | 4,247 | 4,651 | 4,767 | 5,373 |
| Foreign | 32 | 39 | 44 | 47 | 34 | 33 |
| Missing | — | — | 5 | 11 | 156 | 180 |
| GRAND TOTAL | 3,922 | 3,955 | 4,296 | 4,709 | 4,957 | 5,586 |

Due to multiple sources of data for each applicant, the total count per state may exceed the total number of applicants.

| 1995 | 1996 | 1997 | 1998 | 1999 | % Change 1989–99 | % Change 1998–99 |
|---|---|---|---|---|---|---|
| 45 | 40 | 45 | 42 | 49 | 88.5 | 16.7 |
| 404 | 282 | 308 | 276 | 306 | 25.4 | 10.9 |
| 223 | 192 | 201 | 203 | 243 | 111.3 | 19.7 |
| 38 | 70 | 24 | 28 | 13 | 18.2 | -53.6 |
| 257 | 264 | 313 | 343 | 327 | 107.0 | -4.7 |
| 123 | 128 | 132 | 126 | 118 | 100.0 | -6.3 |
| 88 | 74 | 91 | 117 | 116 | 132.0 | -0.9 |
| 247 | 210 | 227 | 228 | 270 | 76.5 | 18.4 |
| 53 | 50 | 65 | 60 | 46 | 91.7 | -23.3 |
| 17 | 9 | 17 | 23 | 16 | 128.6 | -30.4 |
| 44 | 57 | 66 | 66 | 64 | 82.9 | -3.0 |
| 33 | 25 | 27 | 38 | 30 | 650.0 | -21.1 |
| 117 | 126 | 152 | 143 | 160 | 116.2 | 11.9 |
| 396 | 394 | 408 | 427 | 405 | 76.9 | -5.2 |
| 34 | 45 | 43 | 44 | 32 | 100.0 | -27.3 |
| 11 | 9 | 12 | 15 | 16 | -5.9 | 6.7 |
| 174 | 167 | 179 | 162 | 151 | 25.8 | -6.8 |
| 1 | 4 | 2 | — | 2 | — | — |
| 143 | 171 | 193 | 175 | 163 | 77.2 | -6.9 |
| 23 | 102 | 34 | 33 | 32 | 166.7 | -3.0 |
| 178 | 186 | 148 | 166 | 176 | 69.2 | 6.0 |
| 23 | 15 | 18 | 33 | 25 | 177.8 | -24.2 |
| 6,470 | 6,282 | 6,672 | 6,743 | 6,701 | 72.3 | -0.6 |
| 50 | 16 | 14 | 54 | 10 | -68.8 | -81.5 |
| 81 | 203 | 81 | 76 | 70 | — | -7.9 |
| 6,634 | 6,501 | 6,767 | 6,873 | 6,781 | 72.9 | -1.3 |

## Table 5
## Number of Applications per Applicant by Residence, 1999

| State | Applicants | Number of Applicants Submitting One or More Applications | | | | |
|---|---|---|---|---|---|---|
| | | 1 | 2 | 3 | 4 | 5 |
| Alabama | 153 | 113 | 12 | 9 | 6 | 5 |
| Alaska | 7 | 2 | 0 | 0 | 0 | 0 |
| Arizona | 74 | 3 | 2 | 18 | 12 | 8 |
| Arkansas | 36 | 10 | 10 | 5 | 5 | 2 |
| California | 538 | 119 | 34 | 40 | 53 | 47 |
| Colorado | 350 | 282 | 7 | 7 | 11 | 10 |
| Connecticut | 50 | 7 | 3 | 3 | 4 | 2 |
| Delaware | 18 | 3 | 0 | 0 | 0 | 0 |
| Dist. of Col. | 1 | 1 | 0 | 0 | 0 | 0 |
| Florida | 265 | 58 | 31 | 42 | 30 | 19 |
| Georgia | 239 | 112 | 35 | 23 | 21 | 13 |
| Hawaii | 24 | 1 | 0 | 4 | 4 | 2 |
| Idaho | 41 | 22 | 6 | 7 | 0 | 4 |
| Illinois | 263 | 76 | 24 | 37 | 27 | 26 |
| Indiana | 126 | 55 | 16 | 15 | 11 | 9 |
| Iowa | 128 | 109 | 3 | 5 | 3 | 3 |
| Kansas | 118 | 99 | 8 | 2 | 2 | 2 |
| Kentucky | 102 | 69 | 8 | 5 | 8 | 2 |
| Louisiana | 202 | 165 | 12 | 10 | 5 | 3 |
| Maine | 11 | 4 | 2 | 1 | 1 | 1 |
| Maryland | 144 | 31 | 14 | 9 | 14 | 19 |
| Massachusetts | 182 | 81 | 2 | 14 | 12 | 10 |
| Michigan | 226 | 98 | 37 | 23 | 20 | 15 |
| Minnesota | 137 | 71 | 21 | 25 | 8 | 3 |
| Mississippi | 79 | 67 | 2 | 1 | 2 | 1 |
| Missouri | 158 | 142 | 4 | 1 | 3 | 4 |
| Montana | 39 | 3 | 7 | 12 | 10 | 1 |
| Nebraska | 65 | 48 | 6 | 3 | 3 | 3 |
| Nevada | 15 | 2 | 1 | 0 | 2 | 3 |
| New Hampshire | 27 | 8 | 0 | 3 | 1 | 1 |

| 6 | 7 | 8 | 9 | 10 | >10 | Total Applications | Applications per Applicants |
|---|---|---|---|---|---|---|---|
| 4 | 2 | 0 | 1 | 1 | 0 | 270 | 1.76 |
| 0 | 3 | 1 | 1 | 0 | 0 | 40 | 5.71 |
| 5 | 3 | 4 | 3 | 2 | 14 | 482 | 6.51 |
| 1 | 0 | 1 | 0 | 0 | 2 | 112 | 3.11 |
| 34 | 38 | 25 | 21 | 21 | 106 | 3,424 | 6.36 |
| 8 | 10 | 5 | 3 | 1 | 6 | 690 | 1.97 |
| 8 | 3 | 1 | 2 | 5 | 12 | 377 | 7.54 |
| 2 | 5 | 1 | 3 | 0 | 4 | 145 | 8.06 |
| 0 | 0 | 0 | 0 | 0 | 0 | 1 | 1.00 |
| 23 | 11 | 9 | 7 | 11 | 24 | 1,274 | 4.81 |
| 8 | 9 | 4 | 4 | 2 | 8 | 722 | 3.02 |
| 4 | 3 | 1 | 1 | 1 | 3 | 153 | 6.38 |
| 0 | 1 | 0 | 0 | 0 | 1 | 96 | 2.34 |
| 24 | 17 | 5 | 13 | 5 | 9 | 1,087 | 4.13 |
| 6 | 6 | 0 | 3 | 0 | 5 | 404 | 3.21 |
| 1 | 1 | 2 | 1 | 0 | 0 | 195 | 1.52 |
| 4 | 0 | 0 | 0 | 0 | 1 | 174 | 1.47 |
| 4 | 2 | 3 | 0 | 0 | 1 | 219 | 2.15 |
| 2 | 2 | 2 | 0 | 0 | 1 | 309 | 1.53 |
| 0 | 1 | 1 | 0 | 0 | 0 | 35 | 3.18 |
| 11 | 21 | 5 | 6 | 2 | 12 | 744 | 5.17 |
| 9 | 6 | 9 | 3 | 8 | 28 | 869 | 4.77 |
| 12 | 11 | 0 | 3 | 2 | 5 | 653 | 2.89 |
| 4 | 0 | 1 | 0 | 1 | 3 | 314 | 2.29 |
| 3 | 1 | 0 | 0 | 1 | 1 | 133 | 1.68 |
| 3 | 1 | 0 | 0 | 0 | 0 | 210 | 1.33 |
| 3 | 2 | 0 | 0 | 0 | 1 | 150 | 3.85 |
| 0 | 1 | 0 | 0 | 1 | 0 | 113 | 1.74 |
| 0 | 1 | 4 | 1 | 0 | 1 | 86 | 5.73 |
| 3 | 4 | 1 | 2 | 1 | 3 | 148 | 5.48 |

# Table 5 (cont.)

| State | Applicants | Number of Applicants Submitting One or More Applications | | | | |
|---|---|---|---|---|---|---|
| | | 1 | 2 | 3 | 4 | 5 |
| New Jersey | 123 | 18 | 7 | 9 | 5 | 11 |
| New Mexico | 49 | 14 | 3 | 10 | 5 | 3 |
| New York | 306 | 45 | 24 | 27 | 33 | 25 |
| North Carolina | 243 | 133 | 24 | 18 | 25 | 13 |
| North Dakota | 13 | 2 | 1 | 2 | 2 | 3 |
| Ohio | 327 | 241 | 14 | 18 | 11 | 11 |
| Oklahoma | 118 | 82 | 8 | 10 | 6 | 4 |
| Oregon | 116 | 59 | 23 | 7 | 7 | 13 |
| Pennsylvania | 270 | 54 | 21 | 25 | 37 | 29 |
| Puerto Rico | 46 | 13 | 4 | 6 | 4 | 2 |
| Rhode Island | 16 | 9 | 1 | 0 | 1 | 1 |
| South Carolina | 64 | 23 | 7 | 8 | 7 | 8 |
| South Dakota | 30 | 15 | 6 | 4 | 3 | 1 |
| Tennessee | 160 | 104 | 16 | 12 | 8 | 9 |
| Texas | 405 | 214 | 68 | 42 | 26 | 15 |
| Utah | 32 | 3 | 0 | 8 | 2 | 2 |
| Vermont | 16 | 4 | 2 | 1 | 1 | 0 |
| Virginia | 151 | 55 | 21 | 17 | 15 | 10 |
| Virgin Islands | 2 | 0 | 0 | 0 | 0 | 1 |
| Washington | 163 | 76 | 18 | 22 | 8 | 9 |
| West Virginia | 32 | 6 | 8 | 6 | 4 | 3 |
| Wisconsin | 176 | 81 | 34 | 23 | 10 | 7 |
| Wyoming | 25 | 7 | 1 | 2 | 4 | 6 |
| UNITED STATES | 6,701 | 3,119 | 618 | 601 | 502 | 404 |
| Foreign | 10 | 8 | 0 | 0 | 0 | 0 |
| Unknown | 70 | 29 | 9 | 9 | 7 | 2 |
| GRAND TOTAL | 6,781 | 3,156 | 627 | 610 | 509 | 406 |

Due to multiple sources of data for each applicant, the total count per state may exceed the total number of applicants.

| 6 | 7 | 8 | 9 | 10 | >10 | Total Applications | Applications per Applicant |
|---|---|---|---|---|---|---|---|
| 8 | 8 | 9 | 5 | 11 | 32 | 973 | 7.91 |
| 1 | 4 | 2 | 4 | 0 | 3 | 209 | 4.27 |
| 25 | 26 | 18 | 15 | 14 | 54 | 2,005 | 6.55 |
| 11 | 5 | 5 | 0 | 1 | 8 | 668 | 2.75 |
| 1 | 1 | 0 | 0 | 0 | 1 | 62 | 4.77 |
| 10 | 8 | 4 | 5 | 0 | 5 | 690 | 2.11 |
| 1 | 4 | 0 | 2 | 0 | 1 | 247 | 2.09 |
| 2 | 1 | 1 | 1 | 0 | 2 | 282 | 2.43 |
| 32 | 16 | 14 | 11 | 9 | 22 | 1,412 | 5.23 |
| 3 | 4 | 1 | 2 | 2 | 5 | 230 | 5.00 |
| 2 | 0 | 0 | 0 | 0 | 2 | 58 | 3.63 |
| 2 | 2 | 5 | 0 | 0 | 2 | 219 | 3.42 |
| 1 | 0 | 0 | 0 | 0 | 0 | 62 | 2.07 |
| 3 | 2 | 3 | 0 | 1 | 2 | 344 | 2.15 |
| 8 | 9 | 2 | 4 | 2 | 15 | 1,049 | 2.59 |
| 5 | 5 | 1 | 1 | 1 | 4 | 190 | 5.94 |
| 1 | 2 | 2 | 0 | 1 | 2 | 95 | 5.94 |
| 5 | 9 | 2 | 6 | 1 | 10 | 564 | 3.74 |
| 0 | 1 | 0 | 0 | 0 | 0 | 12 | 6.00 |
| 7 | 6 | 11 | 1 | 2 | 3 | 498 | 3.06 |
| 3 | 1 | 0 | 1 | 0 | 0 | 105 | 3.28 |
| 3 | 7 | 3 | 1 | 2 | 5 | 475 | 2.70 |
| 2 | 1 | 0 | 1 | 0 | 1 | 100 | 4.00 |
| 322 | 287 | 168 | 138 | 112 | 430 | 24,178 | 3.61 |
| 0 | 0 | 2 | 0 | 0 | 0 | 24 | 2.40 |
| 1 | 1 | 3 | 0 | 6 | 3 | 246 | 3.51 |
| 323 | 288 | 173 | 138 | 118 | 433 | 24,448 | 3.61 |

## Table 6
## Applicants to U.S. Colleges of Veterinary Medicine
## by Ethnicity and Gender, 1987-1999

| | Year | Total Applicants | Caucasian | Minority* Applicants | African-American |
|---|---|---|---|---|---|
| **Total** | 1987 | 4,758 | 4,106 | 326 | 104 |
| **Applicants** | 1988 | 4,509 | 3,891 | 309 | 110 |
| | 1989 | 3,922 | 3,619 | 303 | 90 |
| | 1990 | 3,955 | 3,639 | 316 | 88 |
| | 1991 | 4,296 | 3,900 | 356 | 100 |
| | 1992 | 4,709 | 4,210 | 402 | 109 |
| | 1993 | 4,957 | 4,300 | 579 | 115 |
| | 1994 | 5,428 | 4,775 | 603 | 132 |
| | 1995 | 6,634 | 5,966 | 567 | 138 |
| | 1996 | 6,424 | 5,426 | 721 | 110 |
| | 1997 | 6,630 | 5,726 | 704 | 132 |
| | 1998 | 6,783 | 5,720 | 745 | 149 |
| | 1999 | 6,695 | 5,648 | 708 | 135 |
| **Male** | 1987 | 2,019 | 1,717 | 151 | 49 |
| **Applicants** | 1988 | 1,827 | 1,551 | 138 | 48 |
| | 1989 | 1,490 | 1,367 | 123 | 30 |
| | 1990 | 1,465 | 1,344 | 121 | 24 |
| | 1991 | 1,507 | 1,349 | 149 | 44 |
| | 1992 | 1,613 | 1,431 | 148 | 36 |
| | 1993 | 1,719 | 1,484 | 208 | 37 |
| | 1994 | 1,810 | 1,575 | 212 | 43 |
| | 1995 | 2,158 | 1,931 | 195 | 40 |
| | 1996 | 2,027 | 1,703 | 227 | 31 |
| | 1997 | 2,005 | 1,739 | 201 | 33 |
| | 1998 | 2,015 | 1,689 | 225 | 43 |
| | 1999 | 1,846 | 1,539 | 198 | 37 |
| **Female** | 1987 | 2,739 | 2,389 | 175 | 55 |
| **Applicants** | 1988 | 2,682 | 2,340 | 171 | 62 |
| | 1989 | 2,432 | 2,252 | 180 | 60 |
| | 1990 | 2,490 | 2,295 | 195 | 64 |
| | 1991 | 2,789 | 2,551 | 207 | 56 |
| | 1992 | 3,096 | 2,779 | 254 | 73 |
| | 1993 | 3,238 | 2,816 | 371 | 78 |
| | 1994 | 3,618 | 3,200 | 391 | 89 |
| | 1995 | 4,476 | 4,035 | 372 | 98 |
| | 1996 | 4,397 | 3,723 | 494 | 79 |
| | 1997 | 4,625 | 3,987 | 503 | 99 |
| | 1998 | 4,768 | 4,031 | 520 | 106 |
| | 1999 | 4,849 | 4,109 | 510 | 98 |

* Minority totals exclude unknown/unreported ethnic identity numbers.

| Hispanic | Native Amer/ Alaskan | Asian/Polynesian | Other | Unreported/ Unknown |
|---|---|---|---|---|
| 141 | 25 | 56 | | |
| 117 | 23 | 59 | | |
| 121 | 23 | 69 | | |
| 122 | 22 | 84 | | |
| 148 | 22 | 86 | | 40 |
| 176 | 43 | 74 | | 97 |
| 180 | 45 | 239 | | 78 |
| 184 | 58 | 229 | | 50 |
| 200 | 42 | 154 | 33 | 101 |
| 233 | 59 | 277 | 42 | 277 |
| 242 | 67 | 189 | 74 | 200 |
| 243 | 75 | 206 | 72 | 318 |
| 226 | 55 | 204 | 88 | 339 |
| 69 | 12 | 21 | | |
| 58 | 12 | 20 | | |
| 58 | 11 | 24 | | |
| 61 | 9 | 27 | | |
| 67 | 11 | 27 | | 9 |
| 77 | 13 | 22 | | 34 |
| 69 | 13 | 89 | | 27 |
| 79 | 21 | 69 | | 23 |
| 70 | 14 | 54 | 17 | 32 |
| 78 | 20 | 85 | 13 | 97 |
| 72 | 23 | 48 | 25 | 65 |
| 77 | 29 | 50 | 26 | 101 |
| 71 | 17 | 50 | 23 | 109 |
| 72 | 13 | 35 | | |
| 59 | 11 | 39 | | |
| 63 | 12 | 45 | | |
| 61 | 13 | 57 | | |
| 81 | 11 | 59 | | 31 |
| 99 | 30 | 52 | | 63 |
| 111 | 32 | 150 | | 51 |
| 105 | 37 | 160 | | 27 |
| 130 | 28 | 100 | 16 | 69 |
| 155 | 39 | 192 | 29 | 180 |
| 170 | 44 | 141 | 49 | 135 |
| 166 | 46 | 156 | 46 | 217 |
| 155 | 38 | 154 | 65 | 230 |

*Table 7*
**Acceptances by Gender, 1995-99**

|  | 1995 | | | 1996 | | |
|---|---|---|---|---|---|---|
|  | *Applications* | *Acceptances* | *Percent Accepted* | *Applications* | *Acceptances* | *Percent Accepted* |
| MALE | 2,158 | 741 | 34.3 | 2,027 | 779 | 38.4 |
| New Applicants | 1,564 | 544 | 34.8 | 1,480 | 584 | 39.5 |
| Repeat Applicants | 594 | 197 | 33.2 | 548 | 195 | 35.6 |
| FEMALE | 4,476 | 1,539 | 34.4 | 4.397 | 1,514 | 34.4 |
| New Applicants | 3,315 | 1,170 | 35.3 | 3,260 | 1,156 | 35.5 |
| Repeat Applicants | 1,161 | 369 | 31.8 | 1,137 | 358 | 31.5 |
| TOTAL | 6,634 | 2,280 | 34.4 | 6,424 | 2,293 | 35.7 |
| New Applicants | 4,879 | 1,714 | 35.1 | 4,740 | 1,740 | 36.7 |
| Repeat Applicants | 1,755 | 566 | 32.3 | 1,685 | 553 | 32.8 |

## Applications, Applicants, and Positions, U.S. Colleges of Veterinary Medicine, 1980-99

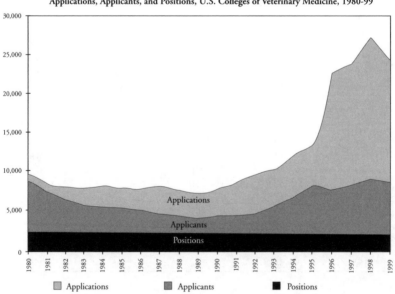

Applications, Applicants, and Positions, U.S. Colleges of Veterinary Medicine, 1980-99

| 1997 | | | 1998 | | | 1999* | | |
|---|---|---|---|---|---|---|---|---|
| *Applications* | *Acceptances* | *Percent Accepted* | *Applications* | *Acceptances* | *Percent Accepted* | *Applications* | *Acceptances* | *Percent Accepted* |
| 2,005 | 665 | 33.17 | 2,015 | 617 | 30.62 | 1,846 | 622 | 33.69 |
| 1,415 | 488 | 34.49 | 1,319 | 424 | 32.15 | 1,172 | 414 | 35.32 |
| 590 | 177 | 30.00 | 696 | 193 | 27.73 | 674 | 208 | 30.86 |
| 4,625 | 1,542 | 33.34 | 4,768 | 1,572 | 32.97 | 4,849 | 1,576 | 32.50 |
| 3,285 | 1,166 | 35.49 | 3,158 | 1,104 | 34.96 | 3,157 | 1,107 | 35.06 |
| 1,340 | 376 | 28.06 | 1,610 | 468 | 29.07 | 1,692 | 469 | 27.72 |
| 6,630 | 2,207 | 33.29 | 6,783 | 2,189 | 32.27 | 6,695 | 2,198 | 32.83 |
| 4,700 | 1,654 | 35.19 | 4,477 | 1,528 | 34.13 | 4,329 | 1,521 | 35.14 |
| 1,930 | 553 | 28.65 | 2,306 | 661 | 28.66 | 2,366 | 677 | 28.61 |

* Does not represent final acceptance numbers

## New and Repeat Applicants, U.S. Colleges of Veterinary Medicine, 1984-1999

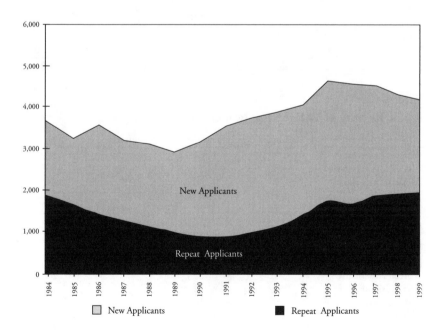

## Table 8
**Ethnic Identity of VMCAS Applicants by Institution, 1999**

| School | African American | Hispanic American | Mexican American | Other Latino | American Indian | Filipino American | Chinese American |
|---|---|---|---|---|---|---|---|
| Auburn | 8 | 18 | 2 | 9 | 5 | 2 | 7 |
| UCDavis | 15 | 23 | 22 | 19 | 12 | 4 | 43 |
| Cornell | 25 | 33 | 14 | 15 | 7 | 3 | 29 |
| Florida | 22 | 32 | 3 | 14 | 5 | 0 | 13 |
| Georgia | 15 | 19 | 3 | 9 | 6 | 4 | 8 |
| Illinois | 16 | 20 | 8 | 12 | 6 | 4 | 23 |
| Iowa | 11 | 23 | 2 | 11 | 8 | 3 | 16 |
| Kansas | 4 | 20 | 3 | 8 | 6 | 2 | 8 |
| Louisiana | 22 | 44 | 11 | 20 | 11 | 3 | 15 |
| Michigan | 24 | 32 | 14 | 17 | 12 | 4 | 23 |
| Minnesota | 20 | 21 | 13 | 12 | 9 | 5 | 18 |
| Mississippi | 3 | 11 | 5 | 8 | 5 | 3 | 4 |
| N Carolina | 27 | 29 | 8 | 19 | 6 | 3 | 13 |
| Ohio | 9 | 16 | 2 | 13 | 3 | 1 | 15 |
| Oklahoma | 1 | 14 | 5 | 7 | 19 | 1 | 3 |
| Oregon | 10 | 26 | 12 | 12 | 11 | 2 | 22 |
| UPenn | 23 | 26 | 13 | 15 | 4 | 4 | 30 |
| Purdue | 19 | 16 | 9 | 17 | 4 | 1 | 16 |
| Tennessee | 16 | 9 | 2 | 4 | 6 | 1 | 3 |
| Texas A&M | 12 | 28 | 12 | 15 | 8 | 2 | 16 |
| VA-MD Reg. | 20 | 16 | 4 | 8 | 4 | 3 | 17 |
| Washington | 10 | 24 | 13 | 14 | 13 | 4 | 25 |
| Wisconsin | 13 | 30 | 14 | 13 | 8 | 4 | 24 |
| U.S. Subtotal | 345 | 530 | 194 | 291 | 178 | 63 | 391 |
| UPEI | 8 | 14 | 5 | 6 | 4 | 1 | 10 |
| Guelph | 0 | 0 | 0 | 2 | 0 | 0 | 0 |
| TOTAL | 353 | 544 | 199 | 299 | 182 | 64 | 401 |

## Table 9
**Ethnic Identity of VMCAS Applicants, 1999**

| Ethnic Identity | Males | Females | Unknown | Total |
|---|---|---|---|---|
| African American | 19 | 64 | 0 | 83 |
| Hispanic American | 36 | 73 | 0 | 109 |
| Mexican American | 11 | 35 | 0 | 46 |
| Other Latino | 13 | 27 | 0 | 40 |
| American Indian | 14 | 32 | 0 | 46 |
| Filipino American | 3 | 10 | 0 | 13 |
| Chinese American | 11 | 50 | 0 | 61 |
| East Indian | 5 | 8 | 0 | 13 |
| Japanese American | 8 | 28 | 0 | 36 |
| Korean American | 10 | 25 | 0 | 35 |
| Pacific Islander | 2 | 2 | 0 | 4 |
| Other Asian | 7 | 16 | 0 | 23 |
| White | 1,138 | 3,168 | 0 | 4,306 |
| Other | 15 | 45 | 1 | 61 |
| Declined to state | 102 | 259 | 37 | 398 |
| TOTAL | 1,394 | 3,842 | 38 | 5,274 |

| East Indian | Japanese American | Korean American | Pacific Islander | Other Asian | White | Other | Declined to State | Total |
|---|---|---|---|---|---|---|---|---|
| 1 | 3 | 5 | 1 | 2 | 505 | 3 | 42 | 613 |
| 6 | 23 | 17 | 3 | 8 | 731 | 20 | 112 | 1,058 |
| 6 | 6 | 13 | 0 | 6 | 944 | 20 | 118 | 1,239 |
| 2 | 6 | 5 | 2 | 7 | 632 | 13 | 56 | 812 |
| 1 | 2 | 5 | 0 | 4 | 670 | 12 | 62 | 820 |
| 7 | 6 | 12 | 0 | 5 | 835 | 12 | 107 | 1,073 |
| 5 | 6 | 6 | 1 | 1 | 797 | 10 | 67 | 967 |
| 2 | 5 | 4 | 0 | 0 | 421 | 8 | 38 | 529 |
| 1 | 9 | 7 | 1 | 5 | 907 | 15 | 73 | 1,144 |
| 6 | 13 | 14 | 0 | 6 | 1,033 | 16 | 103 | 1,317 |
| 3 | 9 | 8 | 1 | 4 | 824 | 13 | 76 | 1,036 |
| 1 | 3 | 3 | 0 | 0 | 315 | 2 | 32 | 395 |
| 3 | 9 | 13 | 1 | 7 | 916 | 12 | 84 | 1,150 |
| 1 | 8 | 7 | 0 | 3 | 555 | 6 | 59 | 698 |
| 1 | 3 | 3 | 1 | 0 | 375 | 6 | 31 | 470 |
| 1 | 19 | 10 | 1 | 4 | 752 | 17 | 87 | 986 |
| 9 | 13 | 16 | 0 | 7 | 1,055 | 20 | 143 | 1,378 |
| 7 | 8 | 6 | 1 | 4 | 748 | 18 | 73 | 947 |
| 1 | 3 | 1 | 0 | 2 | 377 | 7 | 31 | 463 |
| 2 | 8 | 4 | 2 | 8 | 773 | 7 | 58 | 955 |
| 4 | 4 | 8 | 0 | 5 | 800 | 6 | 93 | 992 |
| 2 | 21 | 12 | 2 | 6 | 828 | 16 | 100 | 1,090 |
| 8 | 8 | 8 | 1 | 6 | 1,051 | 17 | 121 | 1,326 |
| 80 | 195 | 187 | 18 | 100 | 16,844 | 276 | 1,766 | 21,458 |
| 1 | 1 | 5 | 1 | 1 | 307 | 10 | 44 | 418 |
| 1 | 0 | 0 | 0 | 0 | 20 | 1 | 5 | 29 |
| 82 | 196 | 192 | 19 | 101 | 17,171 | 287 | 1,815 | 21,905 |

## *Table 10*
## VMCAS Offers of Admission by Ethnic Identity, 1999

| Ethnic Identity | Male | Female | Unknown | Total |
|---|---|---|---|---|
| African American | 7 | 25 | 0 | 32 |
| Hispanic American | 12 | 18 | 0 | 30 |
| Mexican American | 2 | 17 | 0 | 19 |
| Other Latino | 3 | 12 | 0 | 15 |
| American Indian | 2 | 10 | 0 | 12 |
| Filipino American | 0 | 0 | 0 | 0 |
| Chinese American | 10 | 40 | 0 | 50 |
| East Indian | 4 | 6 | 0 | 10 |
| Japanese American | 1 | 23 | 0 | 24 |
| Korean American | 0 | 9 | 0 | 9 |
| Pacific Islander | 0 | 0 | 0 | 0 |
| Other Asian | 5 | 7 | 0 | 12 |
| White | 483 | 1,345 | 0 | 1,828 |
| Other | 0 | 10 | 0 | 10 |
| Declined to state | 50 | 101 | 19 | 170 |
| TOTAL | 579 | 1,623 | 19 | 2,221 |

## Table 11
### Historical Summary of VMCAS Applications and Applicants, 1996–1999

|                                                      | 1995–96 | 1996–97 | 1997–98 | 1998–99 |
|------------------------------------------------------|--------:|--------:|--------:|--------:|
| Full Participating Schools                           | 14      | 13      | 18      | 18      |
| Partial Participating (Required for Non-Residents)   | 4       | 6       | 3       | 3       |
| Partial Participating (Optional for Non-Residents)   | 4       | 4       | 3       | 4       |
| VMCAS Applications (complete)                        | 18,493  | 19,217  | 24,766  | 21,905  |
| VMCAS Applicants (complete)                          | 4,378   | 4,378   | 5,350   | 5,274   |
| Percent Accepted                                     | 28.43   | 29.78   | 31.03   | 31.73   |
| Applications per Applicant Ratio                     | 4.2     | 4.4     | 4.6     | 4.1     |
| REPEAT* VMCAS Applicants                             | 0       | 994     | 1,308   | 1,515   |
| NEW VMCAS Applicants                                 | 4,378   | 3,384   | 4,042   | 3,759   |

* "Repeat VMCAS Applicants" indicates only those applicants who have applied through the service in a previous cycle.

## Table 12
### Number of VMCAS Applications per Applicant, 1999–2000

| | | Offers per Applicant | | | | | | | |
|---|---|---|---|---|---|---|---|---|---|
| Applications | Applicants | 0 | 1 | 2 | 3 | 4 | 5 | 6 | >6 |
| 1     | 1,760 | 1,202 | 558   | 0   | 0  | 0  | 0  | 0 | 0 |
| 2     | 670   | 468   | 174   | 28  | 0  | 0  | 0  | 0 | 0 |
| 3     | 603   | 422   | 152   | 23  | 6  | 0  | 0  | 0 | 0 |
| 4     | 479   | 326   | 115   | 30  | 8  | 0  | 0  | 0 | 0 |
| 5     | 401   | 267   | 90    | 30  | 9  | 4  | 1  | 0 | 0 |
| 6     | 320   | 208   | 78    | 17  | 8  | 8  | 1  | 0 | 0 |
| 7     | 233   | 152   | 48    | 27  | 6  | 0  | 0  | 0 | 0 |
| 8     | 162   | 101   | 32    | 15  | 9  | 4  | 0  | 1 | 0 |
| 9     | 131   | 87    | 21    | 16  | 1  | 1  | 4  | 1 | 0 |
| 10    | 129   | 93    | 18    | 10  | 2  | 3  | 2  | 1 | 0 |
| 11    | 69    | 48    | 10    | 9   | 2  | 0  | 0  | 0 | 0 |
| 12    | 58    | 43    | 7     | 3   | 2  | 2  | 1  | 0 | 0 |
| 13    | 52    | 37    | 6     | 5   | 2  | 1  | 1  | 0 | 0 |
| 14    | 40    | 30    | 4     | 3   | 2  | 1  | 0  | 0 | 0 |
| 15    | 35    | 20    | 7     | 1   | 3  | 3  | 0  | 1 | 0 |
| 16    | 25    | 12    | 7     | 1   | 2  | 2  | 0  | 1 | 0 |
| 17    | 17    | 12    | 2     | 0   | 0  | 2  | 0  | 1 | 0 |
| 18    | 19    | 14    | 5     | 0   | 0  | 0  | 0  | 0 | 0 |
| 19    | 14    | 10    | 2     | 2   | 0  | 0  | 0  | 0 | 0 |
| 20    | 11    | 4     | 2     | 2   | 1  | 1  | 0  | 0 | 1 |
| 21    | 13    | 11    | 1     | 1   | 0  | 0  | 0  | 0 | 0 |
| 22    | 12    | 5     | 3     | 3   | 0  | 0  | 0  | 1 | 0 |
| 23    | 9     | 6     | 2     | 0   | 0  | 0  | 0  | 1 | 0 |
| 24    | 10    | 8     | 2     | 0   | 0  | 0  | 0  | 0 | 0 |
| 25    | 2     | 1     | 1     | 0   | 0  | 0  | 0  | 0 | 0 |
| Total | 5,274 | 3,587 | 1,347 | 226 | 63 | 32 | 10 | 8 | 1 |